PALACE OF ENIGMA

THE MYSTERIES OF BEECHWORTH ASYLUM

Broken Dreams Series 1.5

ASYLUM BOOKS

BROKEN DREAMS SERIES

PALACE OF BROKEN DREAMS
A Brief History of Beechworth Asylum

SPIRITS OF BROKEN DREAMS
The Hauntings of Beechworth Asylum

CONTENTS

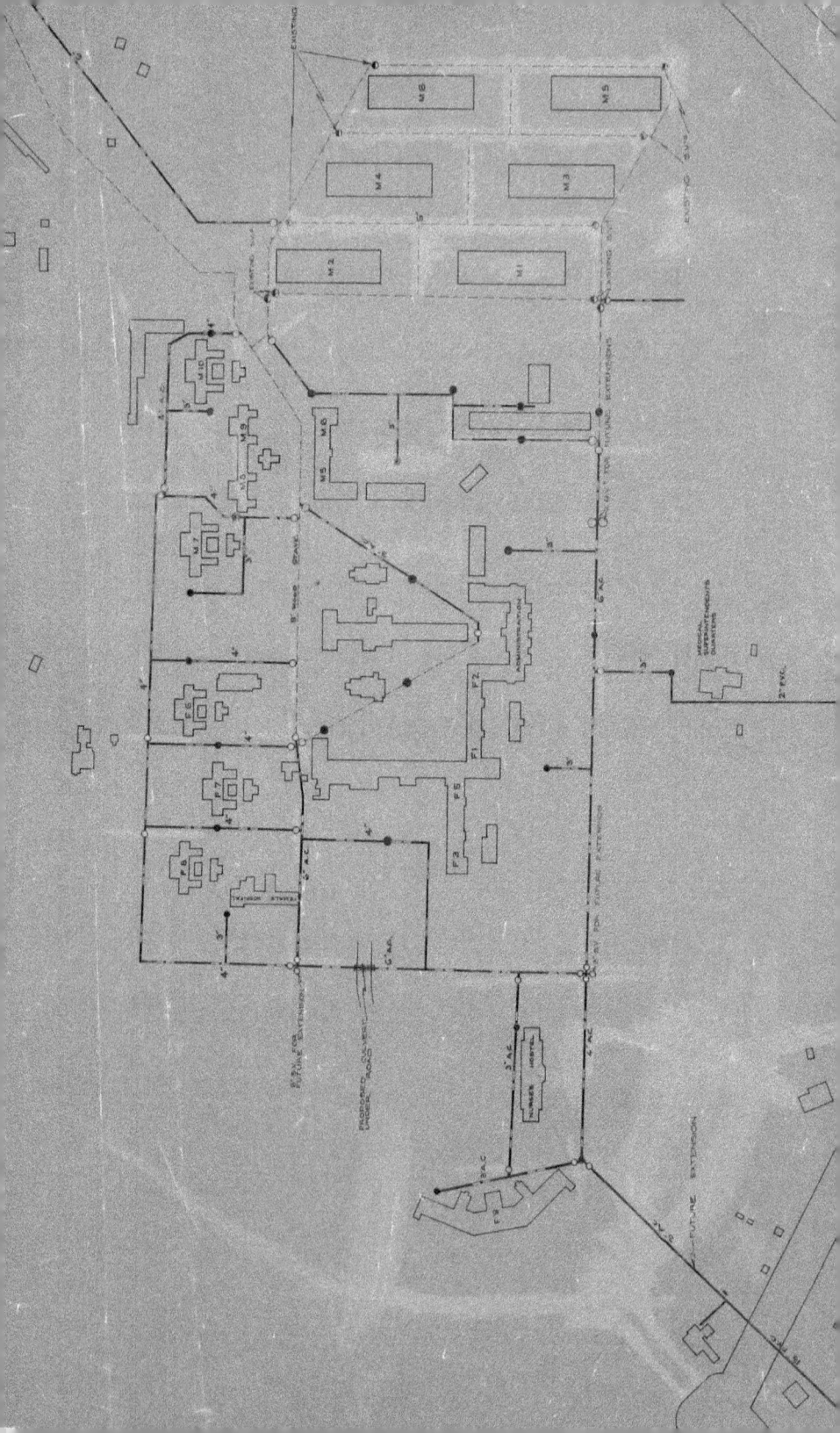

BEECHWORTH ASYLUM: A HERITAGE SITE

The following are extracts from Lovell Chen Conservation Management Plan Review:

"Mayday Hills Hospital is architecturally significant as a particularly fine example of an extensive complex of Italianate asylum buildings dating from the 1860s, and in the case of the cottages, the 1880s. The design is based on the influential asylum at Colney Hatch in England and, in common with other contemporary institutions notably Willsmere in Kew and Aradale at Ararat, displays key characteristic features such as the E shaped plan of the main administration, kitchen and dormitory block with its airing courts, covered walkways, as well as the gatehouse, mortuary and ha-ha wall. The restrained design of the 1860s buildings is attributed to the important Public Works Department architect, JJ Clark." (p.4)

"Mayday Hills Hospital is historically and socially important for its physical manifestation of the changing approaches to the treatment of mental illness in Victoria from institutional confinement to treatment and rehabilitation, and from barracks, through cottages to wards. Beechworth was a key component in a system of nineteenth century asylums which included those at Kew and Ararat. The Mayday Hills Hospital has been crucially important in the social history of Beechworth and has, along with the gaol, contributed significantly to the economic viability and survival of this historically important town. Its size and prominent siting have had an important and long lived social and economic impact on the town and region." (p.4)

"Mayday Hills Hospital is aesthetically important for the beauty of its picturesque setting on a prominent hill among extensive parklands made up of native and introduced trees

1

and shrubs. The curved drive with its avenue of large oaks is particularly noteworthy." (p.5)

Asylum Admission

"Admission to such mental health institutions could be granted in a number of ways:

- Relatives or friends could request an individual's admission as long as they had the appropriate medical certificates from two medical practitioners. With the passing of the Mental Health Act 1959, medical practitioners who had examined an individual could recommend admission to an asylum. The superintendent of the asylum was required to examine the patient as soon as possible after their admission to either approve the recommendation or discharge the individual.
- Two justices could order the admission of an individual who was without sufficient care or discovered out wandering.
- Prisoners suspected of being lunatic could be transferred, with authorization from the Chief Secretary, to an asylum.
- Voluntary admission[1].

Unsurprisingly, it was trickier to get released than admitted. For discharge, eight signatures were needed while only two were required for admission.

Common diagnoses during this time period included:
- Delusional insanity
- Dementia
- Epilepsy
- General paralysis of the insane[2]
- Idiocy
- Inebriation
- Melancholia

-----

1   Voluntary admission: those patients who requested admission for a specified amount of time.

2   General paralysis of the insane: a neuropsychiatric disorder brought on by late-stage syphilis. During the 1800s, it was still considered a psychiatric ailment, due in large part to the psychotic symptoms.

- Puerperal mania[3] .

Up until the 1880s, children deemed especially difficult or mentally challenged were housed with the adult inmates. By 1879, there were close to 600 children housed in such institutions in Victoria. That figure represents a quarter of all inmates at that time."

"During the 1880s, the government deemed it prudent to designate separate buildings to accommodate child inmates." (*Find My Past*)

Asylum Operation

The following are extracts from the *Lovell Chen Conservation Management Plan Review*:

"The... principal members of staff [besides the Superintendent] were a clerk, a dispenser, a matron, and head male and female warders. On opening day some patients were transferred to the asylum from the Beechworth Gaol, and a 'coachload of inmates was brought from Yarra Bend in December [1867]' bringing the total to 71." (p.14)

"Patients at Beechworth and the other government institutions were accommodated in long narrow wards. The beds were arranged in long lines, either side of a central aisle. No screens or partitions separated the beds. The wards were heated by open fires at each end. Furniture was simple, solid and of standard government issue." (p.14)

"Within twelve months, numbers had increased to almost 300, as the asylum became fully operational. Dangerous or violent patients were segregated behind locked doors in isolation cells, where they could be viewed through observation holes. Life at all of the asylums was structured through the use of bells; at Sunbury in 1917, 'no less than 16 bells regulated the sections of the working day'." (p.14)

---

3   Puerperal mania: puerperal refers to the postpartum period, usually lasting 6 weeks after the birth.

"At Beechworth, a range of work was undertaken by the patients, a great deal of which appears to have been on the farm and in the garden. By 1893, the following vegetables and other crops were being produced in considerable quantities: artichokes, beans, beet, cabbage, cauliflower, celery, cucumber, lettuce, marrows, onions, peas, parsnips, pumpkins, radishes, turnips, tomatoes, soup vegetables, fruit, melons, rhubarb, etc., oats, barley, hay, straw, potatoes, green food, and mangold4. Patients also worked in the workshops, where clothing and other items were produced. In 1888, it was reported that 'all the principal articles of clothing issued for patient's use, except boots, were made up in the asylum'." (p.15)

"From the beginning the need for patients to be provided with access to religious services and entertainments of various types was also recognised. Both were specific requirements of all of the state asylums and rates of participation by patients were dutifully reported each year. It is interesting to note that the complex did not originally include a separate chapel... Regular entertainment was also part of asylum life." (p.15)

"Nineteenth century Inspector's Reports[5] provide a list of the ongoing works requirements. Many of the maintenance and repair works could be carried out by the patients themselves, but there was a constant pressure on facilities as the number of patients requiring care rose in the late nineteenth century." (p.16)

"In 1873, extensive additions were made to the Beechworth Asylum. These consisted of the addition of two new subdivisions[6] onto the main asylum building, bringing it closer to completion

---

4   Mangold: beet with a large yellowish root; grown chiefly as cattle feed.

5   Inspector's Reports can be found on the PROV site (https://www.prov.vic.gov.au).

6   A male two storey ward affectionately named 'Bullpit', and a (now demolished) female two storey ward (join can still be seen on outside of and on the top floor of the original women's ward.

of the original design. It was noted in the Inspector's Report of 1873 that when the additions were finished the 'asylum will contain 464 patients'. The Zox Commission of 1886[7] described the additions of 1873 as comprising '19 dormitories and 9 day-rooms,' and as having increased the accommodation 'to a large extent'." (p.17)

---

7   Royal Commission on Asylums for the Insane and Inebriates 1884 – 1886, "[f]requently referred to as the Zox Commission, the Royal Commission was required to inquire into and report upon the state and condition of Asylums for the Insane and Inebriates.

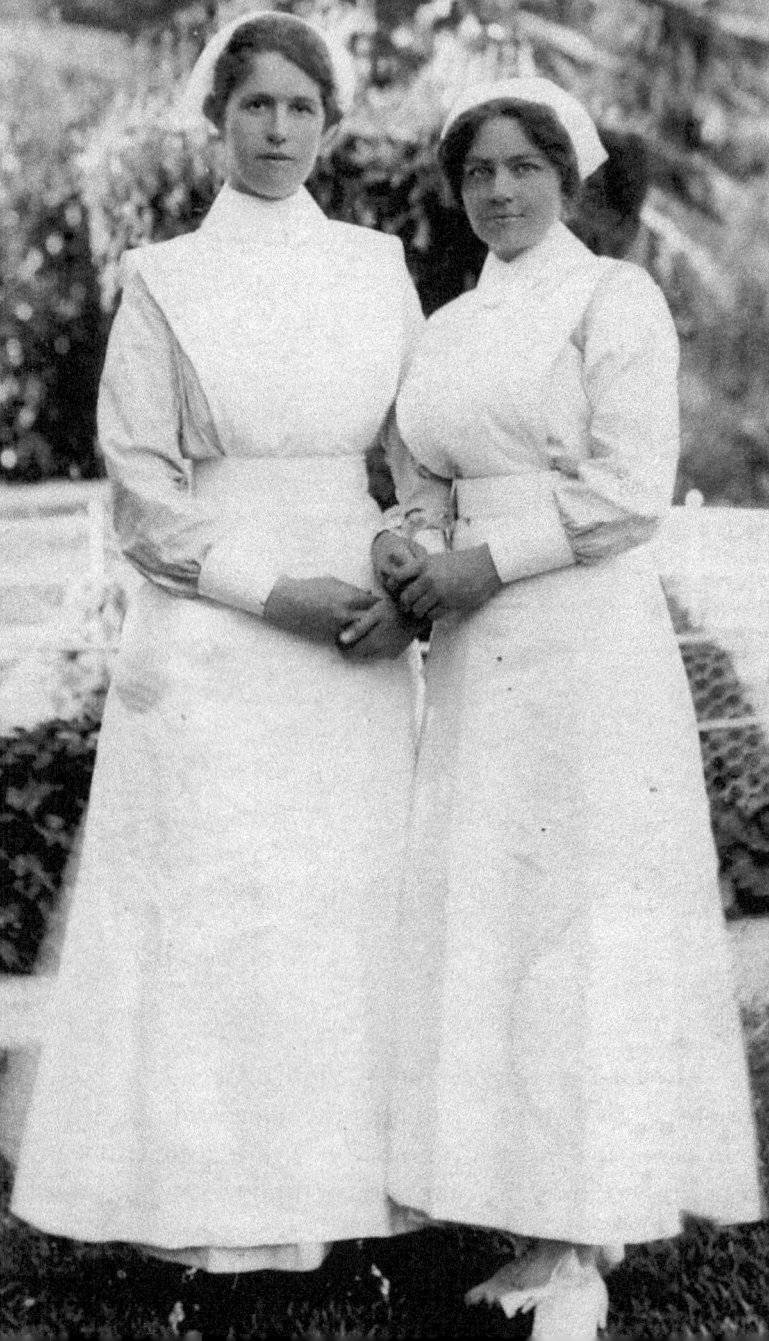

Early Asylum Articles

"The Beechworth Lunatic Asylum"

Ovens and Murray Advertiser Supplement. 23rd May, 1867.

"We give in the present issue, which contains our usual Monthly Summary for Home Readers, an engraving of the Beechworth Lunatic Asylum now all but ready to receive inmates. The sketch is from a photograph by Mr Hall, of Ford Street, Beechworth, and gives an exceedingly full and faithful representation of this fine pile of buildings from the north-western corner of the sunk wall. The foreground will be somewhat altered in time by the removal of the trees which have such a good effect in the engraving but in their place will be English trees and flower beds and handsomely laid out grounds. These grounds will, we presume, in order to be of an appropriate character with the architecture, be in the Italian style of ornamentation, which, with plenty of foliage, fountains, a few statues and a body of water, will be exceedingly suitable to our climate, as well as fitted for the curative purposes, which will no doubt he studied in every single detail of this Institution.

As far as the building itself is concerned it is now completed, and will be occupied within a very few weeks; tenders having been already called for provisions, and orders received by the Governor of the Jail[sic], where lunatics were heretofore locally confined, not to send any more of them to the Yarra Bend Asylum. In this Asylum, situated near Melbourne, all the lunatics in the colony have been hitherto accommodated. Some temporary provision for the security of the patients will have to be made here for the present, as the sunk wall with which it is proposed to enclose the inner grounds has only just been commenced.

It may not be uninteresting to our readers, either at home or here, before describing the new building, to give some idea of the necessity which existed for a more extended system of Lunatic Asylums than had up to this time existed in this colony. The state of the Yarra Bend Asylum was, for many years after the discovery of the gold fields, a disgrace to Victoria. With a mixed, ardent and excited population suddenly thrown upon our shores, their minds already half thrown off their balance by the glowing anticipations which attracted them, together with the sudden possession of wealth by persons, many of whom had not previously enjoyed more than the bare necessaries of existence, it is no wonder that society gave loose to a wild extravagance and recklessness which quickly overthrew the little sense that remained in many weak or ill-regulated minds. Drunkenness and debauchery, too, as a matter of course, lent their aid to heighten a species of almost universal insanity, while the poisonous drugs that in many places were retailed as brandy changed this wide-spread exaltation into downright mania in a great number of instances.

Our jails were full of lunatics or criminals; every day there were accounts brought to the various police stations of men wandering naked with lacerated feet and horror-stricken countenances through the ranges dreading the approach of their fellow men, and vainly endeavoring [sic] to fly from themselves. This is no fancy picture; we are personally aware that there was scarcely a day that information of this kind was not in possession of the police authorities from one part or other of this district.

Horrible mutilations, death from exposure or suicide, were the too frequent endings of those cases, but sometimes the unhappy wretches were coaxed or forced to some human habitation, or being fairly exhausted they doubtfully gave themselves up to the police as the perpetrators of some dreadful and imaginary crime, or for the purpose of seeking protection from some imaginary enemy; but in all cases human reason had, for a time at all events, fled. Undoubtedly drunkenness was the cause of a great deal of this, but as we said, in the extraordinary condition of the colony at that time where every day realities surpassed the wildest dreams of the wildest madman, there was enough to render men susceptible of mental disturbance. The lock-ups and gaols which were then of the most temporary character, without sufficient appliances even for their legitimate purposes, were totally unprovided with accommodation "for these outcasts from human reason"; nor, in very many cases, was a jail the proper place for their custody, and so by degrees, as they were all forwarded to Melbourne, the Yarra Bend became, not merely crowded beyond its very limited capacities, but beyond the possible capabilities of any single establishment. There was not half room, there was scarcely any classification of the inmates — even of the sexes, this was at the time asserted — at all events, if the classification existed in theory, it was not, and could not be carried out in practice; there was little or no supervision over the officers, who were not always chosen for their fitness; there were the short comings of contractors, and in fact all those evils which must result from an overgrown establishment, bad internal government, loose external supervision, and want of means. Great cruelties too were undoubtedly practised, until at length the Press took the matter up, and the public was fairly aroused to the appalling state of things, which had grown up at their very doors. The charitable and humane were astounded at the misery which existed; the thoughtful and scientific, at the absence of all the newest sanitary improvements, and the worldly by the tremendous waste of money which was going on. Argus correspondents, and Parliamentary Committees, and universal surprise and indignation, and a vigorous effort was made to end at once, and for ever, so deplorable a condition of things.

But it was only very gradually indeed, that matters were brought to their present fair state of efficiency. In the first place the buildings were insufficient in size, crowded and incommodious, and the management most unsatisfactory; these evils take time to cure, but they have been cured as far as circumstances would permit. But still it was found that it was bad policy to have under one management so large an establishment, and there were many other considerations which rendered it wise to distribute asylums over the colony. In addition to the already suggested fact, that a more compact institution, which could, in all its most minute details, come under the eye and control of one competent head, there were the additional facts that the expense of conveying lunatics from all parts of the colony was enormous, that the consequences of the rough and exposed mode of transportation were prejudicial to the patients; and, finally, that the almost insensible outside supervision which is exercised by the neighbouring relations and friends of the patients, will be present in the different localities, while it is to a great extent absent in Melbourne.

To show to what an enormous size the Yarra Bend Asylum had grown, we may mention that during 1865 there were no less than 1,270 patients treated there, one-third of whom were females, and that the regular number of beds is over 1,000. The wards are 39 in number, containing an aggregate of 536,310 cubic feet of atmosphere. The cost to the Government for this establishment for the same year was no less a sum than £46,461 6s 8d, almost entirely for maintenance.

Now, it is not an easy matter for one man to govern a regiment of 1,000 soldiers, possessed of their full faculties, and accustomed to a trained and rigorous discipline; how much more difficult, how nearly impossible must it be, then, for one head to overlook and control a thousand human beings who are deprived of their reasoning faculties, and who, although they may in some respects be like children, are in many others as uncontrollable and violent, and far more irresponsible, than wild beasts. It was for these reasons that it was deemed wise to lessen the magnitude of the institution at Yarra Bend, and to establish others in different parts of the country.

The Ovens, Kew, and Ararat were fixed upon as the most fitting localities for carrying out this extension of the system; and in pursuance of this idea the Beechworth Asylum now stands nearly completed, to attest the wisdom, humanity, and liberality of a great colony. As we have already had occasion to give a very full description of this building and its "belongings", we can scarcely do better than partly recapitulate it; but since we have endeavored [sic] to give our readers some idea of what it was intended to be in its complete state, it has already approached its completion, and some of the designs have been altered. The building itself, with the enclosed quadrangles, covers between five and six acres of ground, and contains somewhere about 2,330,000 cubic feet of capacity, independent of the wall, the work-shops, the lodges, and additional quarters still to be erected.

The work already done compares favorably [sic] with that in any other similar under taking in Victoria. We have little hesitation in asserting this, as, even after a building of a like nature and magnitude at Kew had brought reproaches on the contractors of the colony, as well as on some of the Government supervisors of that work, the Beechworth building stood the test of two commissions specially appointed to examine in the strictest manner what had been done here. One of these examinations was in consequence of the delinquencies discovered at Kew, and was one of the most searching character, the walls having been laid bare, and actually taken out to the lowest foundation, at spots chosen at haphazard by the Commissioners themselves.

These "searches" also were quite independent of the ordinary although very strict investigations of the district clerk of works, Mr H. A. Williams; and quite lately the building passed through the ordeal of a visit from the Minister of Works, accompanied by Mr W. Finlay, the travelling inspector. All these authorities did something more than express themselves satisfied with the work done, and so extraordinary an immunity from the slightest blame, where everything is expected, is no doubt due to all concerned.

We would say that the local government supervision by Mr Pickers-gill, and Mr Thomas Williams, the Government inspectors of works, must have been above all praise in so great an undertaking, as where such an amount of public money was involved, the officers representing the State who, without embroiling themselves with the contractors, have earned the approbation of their superiors, must have acted with an unusual combination of knowledge of their business, discretion, purity and vigilance. The magnitude of the building is such as to render it no easy task to convey an adequate impression of it by a pen and ink description. It ought to be thoroughly examined in order to enable any person to arrive at a correct estimation of its importance and vastness. Than the site selected perhaps a better one could not be found in the colony, for the purpose.

Situated on the brow of a hill, about a mile to the south-east of Beechworth, and at an elevation of some hundreds of feet above that township, a view rarely to be equalled, and certainly not to be surpassed in any inhabited portion of Victoria, is obtained from the building. The front faces direct west, or thereabouts, and commands a panoramic view of Beechworth, which admittedly has a very picturesque appearance. In the distance are the deep ravines and gullies, which in every direction surround the metropolitan town of the Ovens, and which are really worth seeing. To the right are heaps of earth caused by the mining operations on Pennyweight Flat, and along the bed of Spring Creek, with sloping vineyards beyond. In the south-easterly direction there is a gradual rise towards Stanley, so that there is nothing to be seen but hills thickly wooded with gum and stringy bark, which, however, promise an abundant supply of firewood for years to come.

The reserve on which the Asylum is situated, consists of about 200 acres of tolerable land for agriculture, and the reserve proposed for the site for an Industrial School is close to it, but the soil there is very good indeed. As it is intended to make the establishment, as nearly as possible, self-supporting, this land will be fenced in and cultivated, the necessary work being performed principally by pauper inmates, who are not so much affected as to render a continual supervision necessary.

Beside agriculture, provision will be made for those unfortunates who are tradesmen to ply their art, and work-shops are being erected with this end, so that a good deal of work of various descriptions will be turned out. Originally, the site on which the building now stands being on the top of a hill, was considerably higher in some places than in others, so that a great deal of cutting and levelling was necessary before the foundations could be dug out. It will be understood that this took some time, when we mention that the cutting done amounted to no less than 42,000 yards.

The first tender of Mr Linacre, which we believe amounted to something like £80,000, was accepted in 1864, and work was commenced on the 16th December, of that year, and ever since there has been, on an average, from 130 to 140 men employed, and on some occasions, the number has reached 250. As for the building itself, as we previously mentioned, the very magnitude prevents a thorough impression being conveyed within the limits of an article, such as the present. The style of architecture employed is the Italian, and in this instance, a design at once pleasing and suitable has been furnished by that much-maligned arm of the Government service, the Public Works Department.

Of course there are minor matters which would be none the worse for a little modification or alteration, and a striking instance of this may be seen in the miserable abortion of a clock tower, which should most decidedly be improved. The front elevation of the main building extends for a distance of 500 feet in a straight line, but the length of the walls is considerably over that. In the centre are towers one storey higher than the other portions of the structure, having an elevation of 54 feet, while the elevation of the other portions is but 46 feet. The main entrances are situated at these towers, one being the entrance to the quarters of the surgeon, and the other the general entrance, through which every person must pass, with the exception of those conveying stores, for whom a separate entrance leading to the store rooms is provided. These towers are square, and about 60 feet apart, the intervening space being portions of the surgeon's quarters, and being nearly the same height as the towers.

The whole is, as it were, advanced from the main building, thus much improving the general appearance. The general

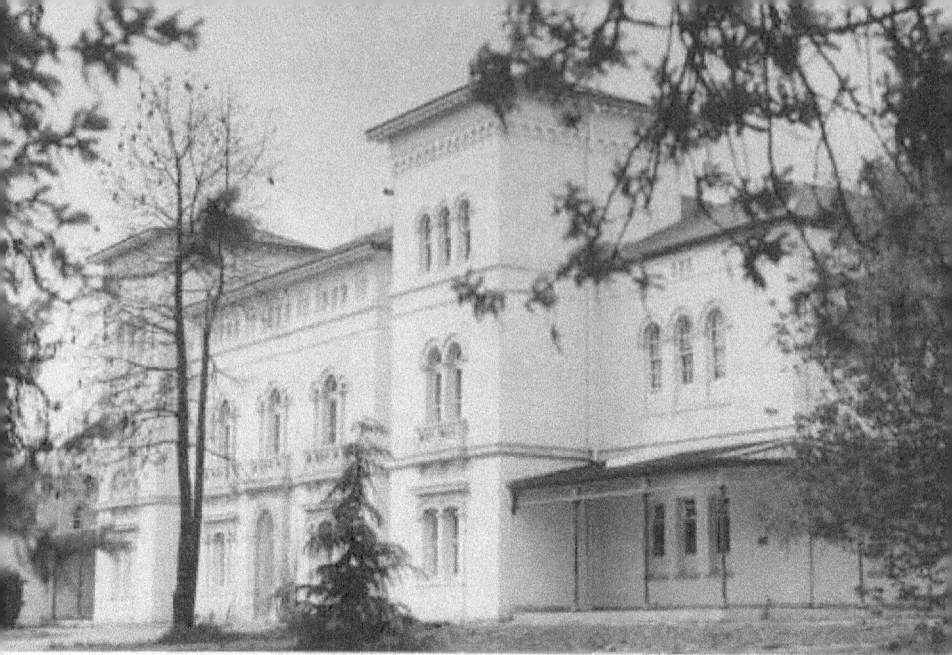

form of the building is that of three sides of a square or nearly so. There are two wings, one 310 feet long, and the other 255 feet. In the centre of the space enclosed by the main building is another branch, containing kitchens, store-rooms, recreation or dining-room, and other space 250 feet in length. The interior of the building is divided into six divisions, three of which on each floor have long corridors, into which all the rooms open. Four of these corridors are 158 feet in length, and about 15 feet in width, and the other two are 125 feet in length, and about the same width as the longer one. A splendid promenade is thus afforded to the inmates, but it is also intended that these corridors shall be used as dining-rooms.

Each of the small corridors mentioned has fourteen single-bedded rooms opening on to it, and there are two smaller corridors in the female division with four each. Out of the total number there are twenty which are lined with boards, and in case of necessity they will be padded for the very violent patients, so as to prevent their doing any injury to themselves. The size of the single rooms in the lower storey is 7ft by 11ft, and 12ft 3in high, and they are exactly similar in the upper storey, with the exception that there is a difference of three inches in the length. The walls are painted to a height of six feet, and above that are coloured. Each room is fitted with every improvement for ventilating purposes, and is provided with one window, containing the usual number of panes of glass, but they are somewhat small, and as they are of thick plate glass it will be impossible to break them, unless with a weapon of some description. Every pane is fitted with an iron fillet. A new idea in the way of shutters is adopted here, and they certainly are of a most handy description, as each shutter balances the other, so that there is no difficulty in completely closing the window over, and this can be done most effectually.

Attached to each division used as a ward are; two large bath rooms, which will afford every facility for thorough ablution. The attendant in charge of each division has two small rooms set apart for his exclusive use, and in these he will take his meals and sleep, so that the greater portion of his time will be with his charge — rather a dreary lot we should imagine. For the inmates who are comparatively harmless there are on both floors large dormitories and day room attached, and a number of these will sleep in the same room, there being a small window which communicates with an adjoining sleeping room for an attendant, who will thus be able to look through occasionally, and acquaint himself with the state of the unfortunates under his charge. Some of these day rooms and dormitories are most-pleasant apartments, and as there is plenty of light and space, and a splendid view from the windows, especially in the upper storey, they seem to be exactly the thing for which they are required. The officer in charge of them has also, in addition to his sleeping room, another room of goodly proportions, also with fine views from the windows in most instances. The same, however, cannot be said with reference to the rooms allotted to the officers in charge of the corridors and rooms opening thereon, for they are rather small.

To each division there is attached a commodious scullery, storeroom, or pantry, which will be fitted with every convenience, so that the work of giving such a large number of helpless beings their meals will be reduced to a minimum. There will also be provided for amusement two reading-rooms and one billiard-room; other pleasure-rooms are also provided elsewhere so that there will be some harmless recreation for those whose intellects are not too thoroughly shattered.

The upper story is almost a fac simile of the lower story, and of course the arrangements will be much the same. In order to prevent any noise or disturbance from the patients walking about on the upper floor, being heard in the lower cells and dormitories, the floors are all double joisted, double floored and "pugged"; that is a portion of the space intervening between the ceiling of the lower divisions and the floor of the upper divisions is filled up with ground clay, which will deaden all sound and prevent it from being heard below. If some such expedient were not adopted, of course the noise of perhaps twenty or thirty people, and some of them with anything but light steps, walking above, would be almost unbearable to the patients below.

The skirtings throughout the building are all of cement instead of wood, and as the material is of the hardest and most approved description, it appears likely that they will be far more durable than wooden skirtings.

The principal means of communication between the ground-floor and storey above will be by a main staircase at the rear of the surgeon's quarters, and this staircase will be a winding or continued rail, one of considerable width. The surgeons' quarters, as before stated, are in the centre of the main building, and comprise the two square towers and intervening space. The rooms are numerous, convenient, and some of them almost palatial in their structure, being extensive, and when well furnished, as they are sure to be, they will be exceedingly handsome.

The front rooms are the most pleasant in the whole building, and the back ones overlook the court yards and back part of the premises. They are situated in the two upstairs floors of the portion of the building indicated, the lower portion around the main entrance being occupied with offices and other apartments necessary for clerical work and for the reception of visitors.

The quarters consist on the first floor, of extensive dining and drawing rooms, six large bed rooms, with dressing rooms attached in some instances, kitchen, scullery, and a large corridor. On the second floor there are eight fine rooms, also part of the surgeon's quarters, so that this functionary will have no reason to complain that due provision has not been made for the reception of so important a personage and his retinue. We also observe a couple of bath-rooms attached to these commodious quarters, and we may say that this important feature in such an establishment is well attended to, as, go where you will, bath-rooms are to be seen, and no doubt their benefit will be thoroughly realised before the asylum has been long inhabited.

There was some doubt whether earth closets would finally be used, as they seem not to have succeeded elsewhere as well as was anticipated, but it was only a question between them and water closets as to the degree of excellence, and the new system has been finally adopted. The contractor for this most important portion of the work is daily expected, and we would fain hope that the Beechworth Corporation and people will not throw away the important lesson about to be taught them in this respect.

We must say that every attention is paid to anything calculated to conduce to the preservation of a good sanitary condition. The position of the site does much towards rendering the preservation of such a state a comparatively easy task, for, perhaps, a more healthy spot it would be difficult to select, at any rate within some hundred miles of it. Every invigorating breeze is caught, and fully enjoyed, while the position of the Asylum, and its elevation, will render it almost free from the hot winds, so devastating in places not so happily situated, and in spite of anything Messrs Paley and Wardell may say to the contrary, we rest satisfied that it is the most healthy spot to be found in the Ovens and Murray districts.

However this is digressing considerably from our subject, so to resume we will now go a storey higher, into a sort of garret place, roughly floored, and with only the rafters for a ceiling. As it is intended that, excepting in cases of very great emergency, this floor shall not be used for anything but a sort of lumber room; this of course matters but very little. Along the sides are arranged a number of 400 gallon iron tanks, which perform a very important part in the scheme for water supply for the building, the bath-rooms particularly, but of that more when we come to the subject.

Along this upper floor is quite an extensive walk, and when the proportions of the building are considered, it will be seen that a quarter of a mile will not be an over estimate of the length of the promenade from the extreme point of one of the wings round to the extreme point of the other, only that an interruption occurs at the main centre building where the surgeon's quarters are located. In some seasons of the year this garret storey would be by no means an uncomfortable place for sleeping in, although too hot for summer time, especially for any person effected on the brain.

Again descending to terra firma, we pass over, under a covered passage, to a building in the centre, of the court yard, and outer first two commodious reading-rooms, one for the males and the other for the females and next to this is a large billiard-room. Adjoining this is a large room 66 feet by 26 feet, which is to be used partly as a dining-room and partly as a recreation room. It is provided with a large orchestra, so that it will be easy enough to provide a pleasant evening's amusement for those of the inmates of the Asylum who are able to appreciate it. Communicating with this room is the kitchen, with a mammoth range, and every convenience required to expedite the cooking operations in an establishment containing, perhaps, three hundred souls, but the cooking will almost entirely be performed in no less than thirteen boilers, of which three are capable of containing no less than 45 gallons each. Large sinks are fitted for carrying oil waste water.

Pantries and other rooms adjoin, and in these a great deal of the food will be prepared for cooking before being taken into the kitchen. The dining rooms for attendants are also under this roof, and it is anticipated that a good deal of the food will also be prepared for cooking in these rooms. At the back of the building are large storing rooms, where all stores of every description for the use of the Asylum will be received, and for which a special entrance is provided, at which nothing but stores will be allowed to pass. This gate — with its lodge and quarters for the gatekeeper, as also a wash-house, we presume, for some of the attendants — will be situated at the rear of the building, and a road from it will lead straight up to the warehouses. Beneath the upper stores very commodious stone cellars are provided for storing wines and other articles of consumption.

The clock tower is also part of this building, but is anything but an ornament. A good view of the clock faces will, however, be obtainable from almost any portion of the court yard, and that of course is a great consideration.

Crossing over again to the north wing, we find large rooms connected with the laundry, principal among which is a

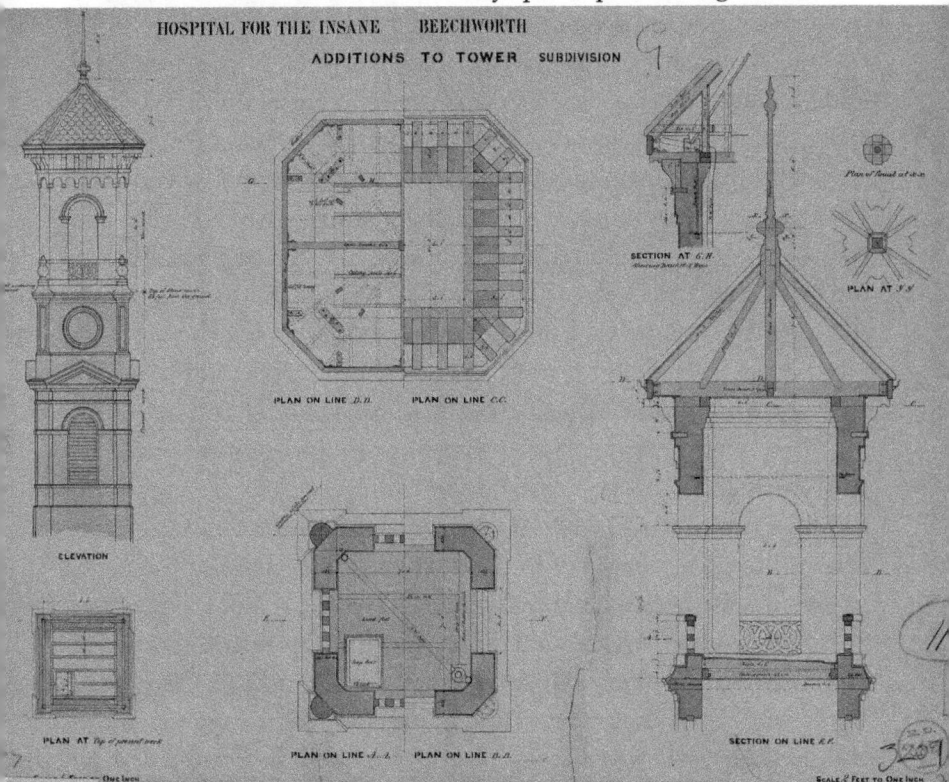

HOSPITAL FOR THE INSANE   BEECHWORTH
ADDITIONS TO TOWER   SUBDIVISION

leviathan wash house, with a height of 25 feet, so that the steam will have every opportunity of rising. Connected with this are sorting rooms, sewing rooms, and last, though by no means least in importance, is the drying room, heated with pipes conveying steam, and fitted with other appliances whereby clothes can be thoroughly dried in the short space of three minutes. Above this are cutting and sewing rooms, and in this again we see evidence of a desire to make the Asylum as nearly as possible self-supporting, for all the pauper female inmates who are not thoroughly incapacitated will take a part in making up the clothes for the establishment.

We now come to the important question of water supply, and when it is considered that the consumption of this element will be about 8,000 gallons per day, it will be admitted that this is a primary consideration. In a building of the size of the Beechworth Lunatic Asylum, it will very readily be seen that an immense amount of water may be obtained from drainage from the roofs, and as the roofs are of slate, it will be of good quality. With a view therefore to economise every drop of this, the whole place is thoroughly spouted, and by a complete system of piping, the water thus kept is carefully stored in seven immense cisterns, each capable of holding about 12,000 gallons. These cisterns are made by digging out an immense hole as it were, and building in it a brick structure nearly of the shape of an enormous egg, which is thoroughly cemented inside and narrowed off at the top to a small hole into which a stone cut for the purpose is fitted, and then a pump is fixed. The size of these cisterns is 23 feet in depth, by 12 feet in diameter, and outside they are thoroughly puddled firm with ground clay. Each one is connected by a large pipe with the next, so that when one becomes full from drainage from the buildings it runs over to the next, and that again to the next, and so on, the last one having an outlet to the back of the reserve.

The cisterns are placed in various places throughout the court-yards, so as to be handy when water is required. Of course, these would be quite inadequate to meet the requirements of the building. A well which will be about 60 feet in depth, will be sunk in the vicinity of the brickyard used by Mr Linacre. As this spot is very much lower than the site of the asylum, and as the well will be carried below the bed of the creek, a supply of water practically unlimited may be obtained from it. But the distance nearly 500 yards, and the elevation to which the water will have to be forced, of course require some extraordinary means of making the supply available. This is proposed to be done by one of Barne's patent hydraulic pumps, a comparatively new colonial invention of great simplicity and extraordinary power. The water, it must be remembered, has to be lifted to the highest elevation in the building, whence it is reticulated as hot or cold water throughout every corner of the Asylum, not for heating, but for the use of the bath-rooms, sculleries, etc.

At the extreme end of the north wing a steam boiler will be erected, from which a one-inch pipe will be laid down to the well, capable of heating from the inside, the enormous pressure of 500 lbs to the square inch. This strength is necessary, as the force used to drive back the water from the well will be air compressed through the pipe to the density of several atmospheres; the water being covered in perfectly air tight. It will be seen that when this enormous pressure is brought to bear on the surface of the water, the power obtained will only be limited by the degree of strength of the materials employed. The water being thus driven by compressed air to the highest and most central parts of the building, a portion is heated by boilers, situated on the ground floor, from which the hot water by a natural law passes upwards, the cold water replacing it. It is then reticulated by pipes whipped with felt, so that the heat will not be distributed till it reaches its various destinations. No universal heating apparatus has been adopted, as in summer the distribution of the hot water would interfere with the comfort of the inmates, and the fireplaces throughout the building are considered fully sufficient in winter. But for a class of patients who require extra warmth there are two suites of twenty rooms — twelve for males and eight for females — at the end of each wing which will be heated by hot water from separate sources.

We had hoped that an effort would have been made, by purchasing some of the many sluice heads of beautifully clear water above the Asylum, to supply this and the other public institutions, as well as the town of Beechworth itself, but there is no doubt the plan adopted will be found fully sufficient for the requirements of the Asylum, itself. The water in the large tanks will be used for drinking purposes only, and will be supplied by common force pumps at each.

Around the whole building are light elegant verandahs and covered ways, leading to the building in the centre of the court-yard. These verandahs are supported by 350 tubular iron posts, which also act as water conductors from the roof, being part of the system of piping for supplying the cisterns with what is caught on the slates. The whole of the verandahs and covered ways are paved with about 40,000 tiles nine inches square. As may be supposed, there was an immense quantity of plastering and coloring [sic] required in such a building.

Supposing that the spaces whitewashed was all made into one patch, it would cover six acres, and, as a good deal of plastering is painted, that, of course, must have been considerably in excess of that quantity. The plastering was sub-let by Mr Linacre, the sub-contractor being Mr Parry, and the same may be said of the painting, but Mr Robinson was the sub-contractor for this.

Much credit we think is due to the gentlemen in charge of the various departments and to Mr Linacre, the contractor. To their universal courtesy we are indebted for a large amount of information which we could not otherwise have laid before our readers. These gentlemen are, besides those already named, Mr Beardall who is in charge of the masons and bricklayers and their portion of the work; Mr Parnham who performs a similar office in connection with the carpenters; Mr Cupit, in charge of the quarries and carrying department; and Mr Glencross who has the receiving and charge of all materials, and the sawmills and brickmaking and we here wish to thank those gentlemen, besides the Government officers, for the courtesy they have shown us.

A few facts in connection with what amount of material it has taken to advance so large a building to its present state will, we are sure, be read with interest. In the first place, as the quantity of bricks required would be so enormous, the contractor determined upon erecting machinery for making them on the ground almost. This was done, and good clay being obtainable within a few hundred yards of the Asylum to the rear, the machinery was erected, and about 3,250,000 bricks have been supplied.

The hardwood required was also cut by the same machinery as grinds the clay and the wood and bricks were delivered by means of a wooden tramway almost at the scaffolding. Tiles were also made for paving the verandahs, and of these somewhere about 40,000 were required. Of granite, 22,000 cubic feet was used for the foundations and footing walls, and of rubblework there has been about 62,500 cubic feet. There is more than half a mile of verandah and covered way, in which 350 iron supports are employed. About 250,000 feet of hardwood have been used, and of soft wood the quantity has been enormous, but no exact return can be furnished. It will be seen that there must have been a great quantity when the carriage from Melbourne has exceeded 1,000 tons.

There is in the building 30,000 feet, or about half a mile of granite base course. Of the work we have attempted to describe, that is of the main building itself and the reservoirs, everything has been completed except the baths, the earth closets, the pipes for reticulation, and a few other small items but a great deal yet remains to be done before the undertaking can be said to be finished.

In the first place one of the most important features in the whole plan — namely, a sunk wall — has only just been commenced. There are also yet to be built two lodges, one at the main, the other at the back entrance, and divisional walls for the purpose of classification. The sunk wall will be thirteen feet high on the inside, with what military men would call a barbican within five feet of the top on the outside. Owing to the unevenness of the ground, these heights must be accomplished by cutting away the earth in some places and filling in at others. The object of the sunk wall is of course to give the patients an uninterrupted view, and it will enclose about 20 acres, being

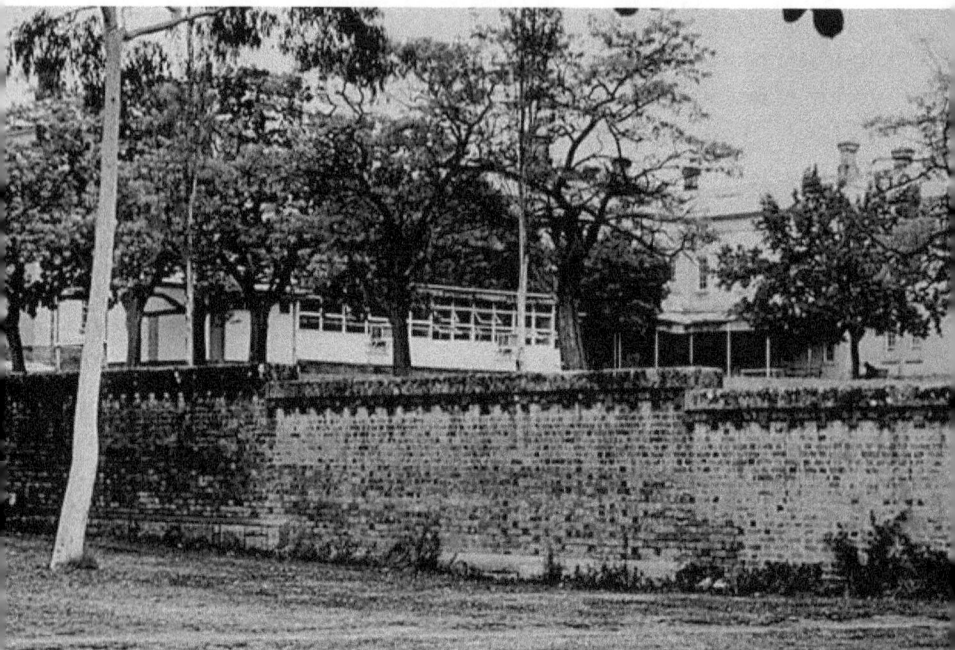

about 1000 feet square. It will be curved with a handsome sweep to the front of the building, so that the central or official portion of the building may be said to be outside it. Besides this entrance, through which both patients and visitors will be admitted, there is none other to the inner enclosure, except a gateway for the necessary goods and provision traffic directly at the back. The contract for the wall is necessarily estimated on a schedule of prices, as it was impossible to calculate beforehand the quantity of rock that would be encountered; but the walls, lodges, work-shops, and outside fence will not cost much less than £25,000.

At the main entrance, which will be at the outside enclosure, in a right line with Camp Street, will be erected a very handsome two storey lodge. Immediately inside this, two avenues will diverge, one going to the main front, and the other to the rear entrance for the heavy traffic. The outside fence will be of sawn timber and six foot palings, and will be nearly 2¾ miles long, enclosing about 200 acres. The outer portion of the reserve will in time be laid out in pleasure grounds, flower plots and kitchen gardens for the amusement and use of the institution.

The whole is intended for the accommodation of 220 patients, that at Ararat being intended for about the same number, and Kew 538. The original reduced contract for the building amounted to £76,096 18s, with an additional charge for extras of £5413 11s. The lodges and work-shops will cost £7,622 9s 4d, and we estimate the wall and fencing at about £16,000 more. If we add the contract for furniture £2029 4s, we will obtain a total of £107,982 2s 4d, surely a princely sum for a humane and noble purpose.

Feeble as our description of so vast a design necessarily is, it may convey some faint conception of the extent and importance of this great undertaking, but it will give no idea of the feelings which it arouses in the mind of the spectator. He, indeed, will he struck by the beauty, elegance, and magnitude of the building but he will also be filled with sentiments of tender pity, when he reflects on what scenes are to occur here, what melancholy spectacles, what heartrending separations, what hopes, perhaps for ever shut out — yet with sentiments of gratitude also for the sufferings that are here to be alleviated, for the loved ones to be restored whole to yearning bosoms, and for the eternal mercifulness of a good God.

Note. — Since the above was in type, we find that Barnes' hydraulic pump is not worked by atmospheric air, as we supposed. The active power appears to be water. The water is forced down the one-inch power pipe by means of a three throw pump, worked by steam power. The action of the water is similar to that of steam, being worked by a slide valve, the power thus applied, raises and lowers a piston in a cylinder, and at each stroke the water is driven up the three-inch main."

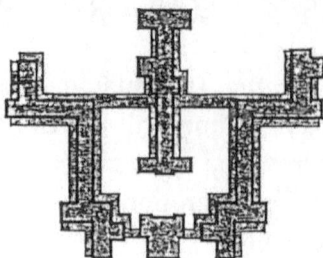

ARARAT LUNATIC ASYLUM

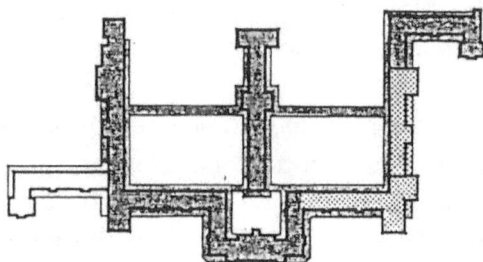

BEECHWORTH LUNATIC ASYLUM

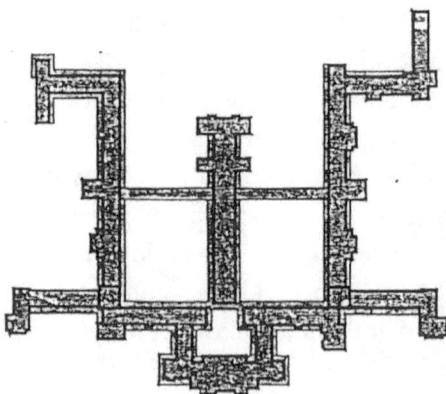

KEW LUNATIC ASYLUM

An excerpt from Glimpses of North-Eastern Victoria, and Albury, New South Wales by Rev. W. M. Finn:

"My readers will be much astonished to learn that one of the noblest buildings in Victoria is the new Lunatic Asylum at Beechworth. This might well be styled the Palace of the Insane[8]. It was during the last O'Shanassy Ministry's term of office that Parliament unanimously resolved to meet the want of room for the rapidly increasing number of the insane, one of the results of which is the imposing Lunatic Asylum at Beechworth. The plans of the building came from the Public Works Department, under the supervision of W. W. Wardell, Esq., Inspector General of Public Works. The building, as regards general design and utility, reflects honour on the department. It occupies one of the most commanding aspects as you enter the town. When it has to be recorded that this building has cost over £100,000, some estimate of its vast proportion may be guessed at.

It is worthy of remark that when a Royal Commission were selecting the site of the building in question they unanimously decided it should be at the head of a gully, which, though unknown to them, was christened by the diggers "Madman's Gully." How strange that in 1854 such a name was given to it, and still stranger that in 1867 a building of such magnitude, and solely devoted to the mad, should rear its head in the very spot. Perhaps those who know whom the initials W. M. F. represent will admit that I have a presumptive right to speak with some weight of authority on Lunatic Asylums. As a visitor of many years standing to the Metropolitan Asylum at the Yarra Bend, my intimate knowledge of the insane will be of value to me in speaking descriptively of the Beechworth Hospital for the Insane.

The new Asylum at Beechworth is quadrangular, built of brick, cemented, and is surmounted by a graceful tower. In the

8   "Palace of the Insane" is the phrase that inspired the title for our first book, *Palace of Broken Dreams*".

27

centre of the wings is situated the superintendent's and staff officers' quarters. The Asylum was opened for the reception of patients in 1867, and Dr. Dick[9] was and is the first superintendent. He was for several years at the Yarra Bend, and is a gentleman whose general kindness and suavity of, manner in many ways fit him to be the occupant of his present office. Dr. Dick stands well with his subordinate officers, and even the poor demented patients are ever ready to smile at his approach. I had a practical illustration of this when I several times accompanied Dr. Dick on his daily rounds through the institution. Mr. D. C. O'Connor[10], a gentleman favourably known in the Yarra Bend, is the steward and chief clerk, and from what I can learn is deservedly popular in the discharge of that office. Indeed, he is most assiduous in the performance of his duty. The head attendant is Mr. Coakley[11], and the matron Miss Bridget Dunne[12], who were both transferred from the Yarra Bend. To those who know them, it is needless to remark that both are fulfilling their allotted duties with credit to themselves, and with the warm approbation of their superiors. Indeed, all the attendants, male and female, are now winning laurels for themselves by their assiduity.

At first, things did not go along so smoothly in this Asylum, but now that the "wheels of work" have become more free by time, things have settled down to a more satisfactory line of action. When the up-country Asylums were opened in 1867, the principal officers and attendants were taken from the picked staff of the Yarra Bend Asylum. It should be mentioned that "political influence" in some cases overruled the above arrangements, much to the annoyance of some who had indisputable claims on a department which they had long and faithfully served. The average number of patients in Beechworth Asylum is 290. Their health has been remarkably good, which speaks well for the

9   Thomas Dick, Superintendent, 1867-1877.
10   Daniel O'Connor, Clerk and Steward, 1867-1894.
11   John Coakley, Head Attendant, 1867-1873.
12   Bridget Dunne, Matron, 1867-1872.

salubrity[13] of the district. For the amusements of the patients a large music hall is in the centre of the square, and in this on each Wednesday evening some entertainment for the delectation of the inmates is held. On Sundays the asylum is a great rendezvous for pleasure-seekers from Beechworth. Indeed, it is not too much to say that it has become quite the favourite resort of those who can have a few hours' "outings." A good permanent supply of water is a desideratum that is much felt, and the Government, if only for the sake of the cleanliness of the establishment, should supply it at any cost... The extreme cleanliness of the Beechworth Asylum, coupled with the cheerful appearance of the patients, are things to be highly commended. The Inspector-General of Lunatic Asylums pays four visits annually to Beechworth, and he invariably has to report most favourably of the working of the institution. Those whose friends are unfortunately insane can comfort themselves with the reflection that, in all the Victorian Asylums, nothing will be left undone to win them back once more to sanity, or else alleviate their afflictions." (pp.24-26)

---

13 Salubrity: healthfulness - the quality of promoting good health.

"A Run Through Beechworth Lunatic Asylum"
Ovens and Murray Advertiser.
6th June, 1903. p.11.

"A lunatic asylum, like a prison, is one of those estimable public institutions which we all admire most at a distance, but which very few of us care to become too intimately acquainted with. The spectacle of hundreds of our fellow human beings with brains turned topsy turvy, and with mental and moral faculties all deranged and more or less perverted, is not exactly calculated to inspire the beholder with feelings of delight, unless it be in that narrow and restricted sense in which Burke uses the word — the delight we experience at finding ourselves exempt from the horrors which we contemplate and unenveloped by the misfortunes which we deplore. There was a book once published which endeavoured to show little boys what a world without law would be like. In this world nobody ever knew for certain what was going to happen next. The sun might rise in the morning, but that was no guarantee that it would set in the evening; or it might rise in the west, and set in the east; or it might not set at all. If you threw a ball into the air, there was no particular reason for supposing that it would come down again; it might explode, or it might turn into an apple. Why not? Everything depended on chance. Now some such uncertain and uneasy feeling which a world of chance would produce in the minds of its denizens takes possession of a visitor who goes for the first time through an asylum for the insane. The moment the outer gates admit you into the ground you prepare yourself to be surprised at nothing. You are entering an inverted world, a world of caprice, a world without law, and a world which, if left to itself, would soon be a worse pandemonium than Dante ever imagined.

A CONTRAST.

But — and here is the weak point in the analogy — it is not

left to itself; no, not for a single moment. And that makes all the difference imaginable. Over the elements of disruption and chaos sits a reigning intelligence, a superintending system of order which co-ordinates and subordinates everything to certain definite and specific ends. For you must know that a first class modern Lunatic Asylum serves quite a variety of purposes. In the popular mind it is merely a place for the isolation and safety of the dangerous. It is this; but it is also a great hygienic hospital for the restoration of the insane to physical and mental health; it is a house for moral and physical education; a school for elementary, artistic, scientific, literary, and even religious training. It is a place of numerous and orderly activities, of homely industrial occupations, where the heads and the hands of the inmates are called into systematic, healthful and daily exercise. So much has been said of late in criticism of our Victorian asylums — and I am not going to say such criticisms are uncalled for, since I am not in a position to judge — that the public, which takes but a very languid interest in these institutions, is in danger of underestimating their value to the community, and of failing to appreciate the great sanitary work that goes on silently within them. To understand this work it is necessary to compare the position of the lunatic of to-day with his position a hundred years ago even. In nothing are the humanising tendencies of modern civilisation more apparent. For many centuries the lunatic, the idiot and the imbicile [sic] were permitted to wander about clotheless [sic] and homeless, the sport of the wanton and wicked thoughtlessness of children. The frantic and furious were chained up in loathsome dungeons and exhibited for money like wild beasts. Even where any attempt was made to confine them, they were huddled together without regard to their habits in cells not fit to keep pigs in. The lash was systematically used, and was recommended by high authorities. The inmates were often killed by the ignorance and brutality of their keepers. Monomaniacs[14] became, according to circumstances, the objects of superstitious horror or reverence. They were regarded as

---

14 Monomania: pathological obsession with one idea or subject.

possessed with demons, and were subjected with every token of degredation [sic] to priestly exorcisms, or were cruelly destroyed as wizards and witches.

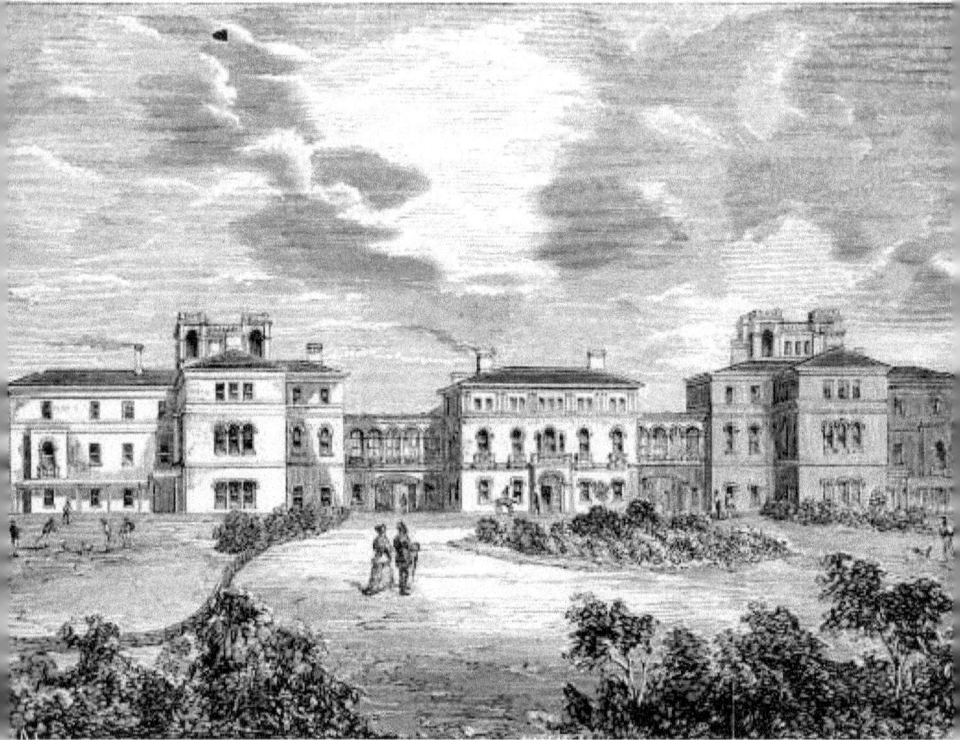

At other times they were made the tools of designing and ambitious men and as inspired instruments of the Deity, became the leaders of revolutions and revolts.

THE OUTER ASPECT.

To form anything like an adequate idea of the striking contrast presented between this dreadful state of things and that obtaining now, it is worth your while to take a stroll through some well-equipped modem asylum like that at Beechworth.

This excellent institution represents, I believe, in a fairly good degree, the most approved and up-to-date treatment of the insane. At least, that was the impression left upon my mind after availing myself of an opportunity, kindly offered me by

Dr. Samson[15], the superintendent, of going through it the other day. The first thing that arrests the visitor's attention — for I suppose my experience in this respect is the common one — is the magnificence of the buildings and the picturesquesness [sic] of the general surroundings. It is not too much to say that the Beechworth Lunatic Asylum is the most prettily situated and the most attractive looking of any public institution in Beechworth, and this is no accident; it is a matter of deliberate design. In the building of an asylum for the insane, two supreme objects are kept steadily in new. The first of these is to make the place as little like a prison as possible, and to carefully eliminate everything in its appearance suggestive of compulsory confinement, compatible with the safety of the inmates. The second point is to secure the best possible sanitary conditions. Both these fundamental conditions are fulfilled in a high degree at Beechworth. Situated at an altitude of 2000 feet above the sea, embowered in pines and eucalypti, with highly-cultivated gardens and fields immediately around it and a magnificent prospect on all sides in the distance, it is hardly possible to conceive of a more favorable [sic] location for the successful treatment of the insane, whose condition is enormously influenced for good by bright and cheerful surroundings and by a pure and tonic atmosphere. The entrance suggests some fine old park; and the clean-shaven lawn, with its pretty border beds of bright flowers, its noble fountain, its rich display of choice conifera, and its varied ornamental shrubs and ferns and grasses make up altogether a scene of floral luxuriance such as I have seldom seen outside of England. It certainly forms a very beautiful setting for the Asylum itself, whose grey stuccoed walls with their slate-covered roofs rise in a shapely pile out of a very appropriate environment. At the Superintendent's room, which over-looks the entrance, I met Dr. Samson who, however, had just previously met with an accident, which had the unfortunate effect of depriving me of his professional experience as a cicerone[16] in my progress through the building.

15   Henry Samson, 4th Superintendent, 1896-1905.

16   Cicerone: a person who conducts and informs sightseers; a tour guide.

However, he did the next best thing possible in the circumstances, he consigned me to the care of his chiefs of staff. Mrs. Short[17], the lady superintendent, was the first to take me in hand, and with her for my guide, I commenced at once a tour of the female portion of the institution. The Asylum is divided into two large rectangles; that on the left of the main entrance being devoted to female, and that on the right to male, patients. These two wings or sections are in all important respects a facsimile of each other. There were 398 female patients in the institution at the time of my visit, and about the same number of males. This represents as large a number as the Asylum will conveniently accommodate. This army requires for its efficient superintendence [sic] some 42 male and about 82 female attendants.

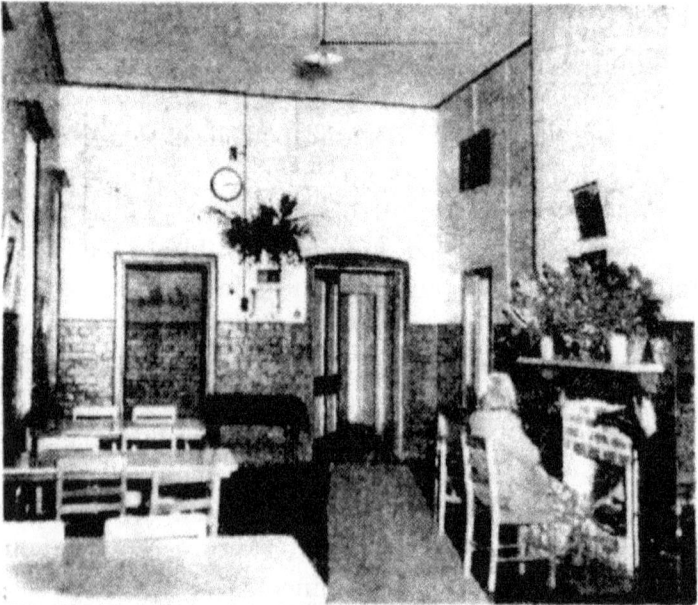

IT WAS COLD OUTSIDE but an elderly, grey-haired patient sat in comfort by a blazing log fire.

17   At the time this article was written, there was no permanent appointment. The staff register has Maria Short listed as the acting matron. Short went on to become the 8th matron, 1907-1923.

THE VIEW WITHIN.

Passing, then, with my guide through a doorway to the left, we enter a long; and well-lighted corridor, which serves the double purpose of a dining and sitting room. The bright, polished saffron-colored [sic] tables standing down the centre, and the substantial wooden chairs to match, combine with the numerous neatly curtained windows to give the room a bright and cheery aspect. And everything from floor to ceiling was scrupulously clean — even to the very air itself. There were no superfluous articles of furniture, but everything was arranged on an intelligent plan, and with a view to combining comfort with the utmost cleanliness. The same remark applies to the large and well-lighted dormitory adjoining. Nothing, I thought, could exceed the uniform neatness of each several bed [sic], standing side by side at equal distances from each other, with their snow-white pillows and carefully-turned counterpanes. At the extremity, a small brass-encircled aperture in the wall reveals the position of the night attendant's room, immediately adjoining, and the means by which she is able at all times to see and to communicate with the next compartment without of necessity going into it herself. This section, the Superintendent informs me, is occupied by patients suffering from the more acute stages of disease. The making of the beds and the domestic work generally is largely carried out by the patients themselves, whose minds have to be withdrawn from dangerous and morbid reveries and their faculties to be employed, where possible, in useful and homely exercises. A flight of stone stairs leads to which is a repetition of what I have described an upper story. Again we have the same characteristics — scrupulous cleanliness, airiness, neatness. The afternoon being warm and sunny, the patients are mostly out of doors — at least, those who are not at work— and from an upper window we get a good view of one of the airing courts outside. This court is an open space flanked by spacious and well lighted verandahs and well sheltered by surrounding trees. In the centre is a large wooden rotunda, which forms an excellent shelter from the afternoon sun. Here a crowd of poor creatures are taking their daily exercises — some are striding aimlessly about, some talking incoherently to themselves, one or two lying asleep on their backs in the warm sunshine, but most of them sitting motionless on the rotunda seats, their Coarse blue shawls drawn closely over their hatless heads or thrown loosely over their shoulders. There they sit day after day, silent and morbid, noticing nothing and caring for nothing. They rarely ever notice or speak to each other. The mind — or what was once the mind — is obliterated; the emotions and passions are gone. They have no desires, no hatreds, and no affections; are docile and passive, without power of thought or power of will. Under some paroxysm[18] of excitement, they will occasionally make an apology for a stir, but the paroxysm over, they lapse once more into a dreary monotony of stupor. This is dementia, that saddest form of insanity — oftentimes the sequel to other phases of mental disease — and representing the gradual and total decay of all the faculties till mere oblivion is reached — sans[19] teeth, sans eyes, sans taste, sans everything. Proceeding, we pass through other corridors and other dormitories equally clean, equally well lighted, and equally well ventilated, stopping here a moment to notice a nicely-arranged scullery and there a well-appointed bathroom. The thing is beginning to become a little bewildering, when we reach the cosily furnished day-room of the female hospital[20]. This suggests the well-furnished sitting-room of a private house. Here the beds are a trifle lower for the benefit of the feeble and convalescent; but a pleasant and neatly-attired attendant — whose name I happen to forget — informs me, with pardonable pride, that she has but one patient in the hospital, and that there has not been a single typhoid case during the whole of the summer — a fact which hardly

---

18 Paroxysm: a sudden outburst of emotion or action: a paroxysm of laughter.

19 Sans: without.

20 Possibly the female infirmary. Two cottages on the female side were demolished and it is believed that one of these was the female infirmary.

occasioned me surprise. In this region dwell the more intelligent and amenable patients — for they have to be carefully classed — and the rooms become more home-like, the walls more regularly hung with paintings and drawings. The tables, too, are provided with magazines, periodicals and newspapers. There are flowers, and, if I remember rightly, even a singing bird or two. The meals are regular and, I am told, sufficient, and there are various table amusements, such as chess and cards, suited to the taste and

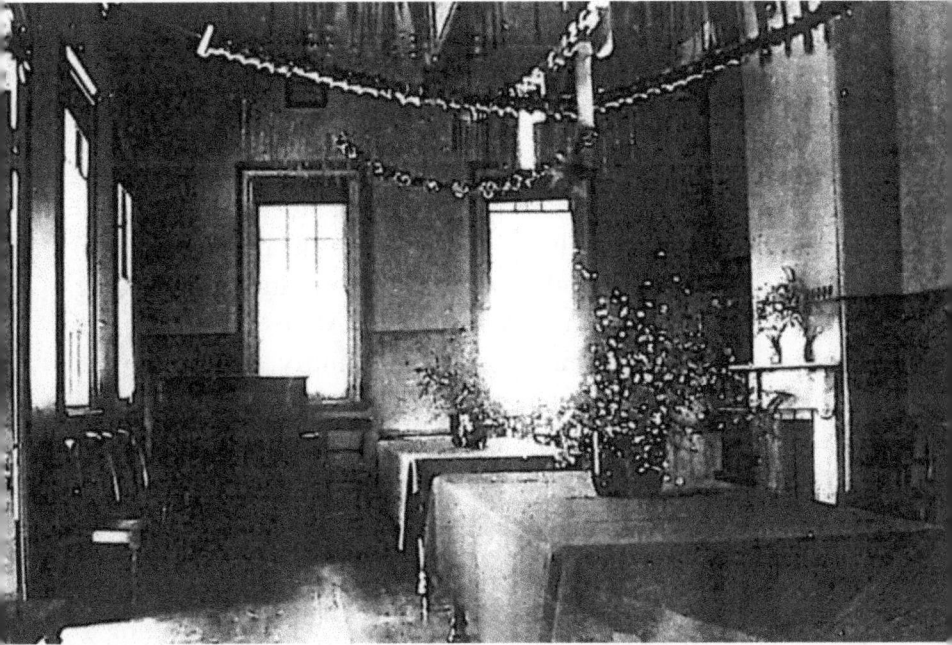

capacity of those who take part in them. The aim is to make the patients feel happy and contented in some purpose which carries the mind away from the subject of their disease, and which is adapted to the varying phases of their malady. To attain this end the better in certain selected cases, there are several nicely built and neatly furnished cottages in a secluded part of the premises. The idea seems to me to be an admirable one every way, but of course it has its limitations with regard to use. It is obviously unsuited to the helpless and the wilder spirits, who would have too much scope for mischief, or who would require too much and too close supervision. On our way to and from these cottages we pass through the interior rectangle, which is provided with a good lawn tennis court, and on which the patients, or such of them as are able, are induced to occasionally play.

THE INDUSTRIAL LIFE.

But while ample provision is made for amusement and recreation, the inmates are encouraged in habits of industry. Thus there are workrooms, in which the women sew and knit and embroider. In one of these I saw quite a small host of workers sitting close together on forms, each with her bit of work upon her lap, and her needle in hand, whilst Miss Collier[21], the experienced tailoress in charge, stood up at a table loaded with fabrics, cutting out and directing her half-witted, and, I should imagine, her sometimes rather unmanageable subordinates. This is the clothing manufactory of the establishment, the material being purchased in Melbourne and made up by the patients, who in this and many other ways assist to reduce the working expenses of the asylum to a minimum. Almost adjoining the workrooms is the washing-house and laundry. This is a scene of great activity, as may be gathered from the fact that nearly a million — or is it ten million — articles of clothing pass through the tub every year. Here I found Miss Doyle[22], the head laundress, moving busily about among a crowd of assistants, who in steam and water were sorting and wringing and drying and ironing and folding a never-ending procession of things that were passing through the mill. "And yet they say we have no-thing to do up here!" said Miss Doyle, a little disdainfully, as she saw my eyes wandering in astonished gaze over a complexity of steam-driven washing and wringing machines, and other accessories too numerous to mention. I said then what I say now, that Miss Doyle is undoubtedly the hardest worked official at the asylum, and if ever I have my way I shall make her the highest paid officer in the establishment, with the man who does the post-mortem examinations next, and the rest practically nowhere. In this way I shall hope to convince Miss Doyle that there is at

---

21 Ellen Collier, Female Tailoress, 1894-1907.
22 Mary Doyle, Head Laundress, 1892-1922.

least one person who holds to the opposite opinion. Just across the open drying yard is the well-appointed blacksmith's shop, where Mr. Oates[23], the engineer, and his assistant, Mr. Rattray[24], have their business quarters. Mr. Oates, who now takes me in hand, shows me over the two adjoining boiler sheds, as well as over the fine engine house where the motive power for the various mechanical operations, as well as the steam for heating, cooking and laundry purposes is generated. He also explains the details of some important engineering improvements he has recently effected in the bathrooms, which have resulted in the more efficient and economical use of water there. Then we pass into the large kitchen where Mr. Christie[25], the cook in charge at the time, is busily heating some five huge copper cauldrons in

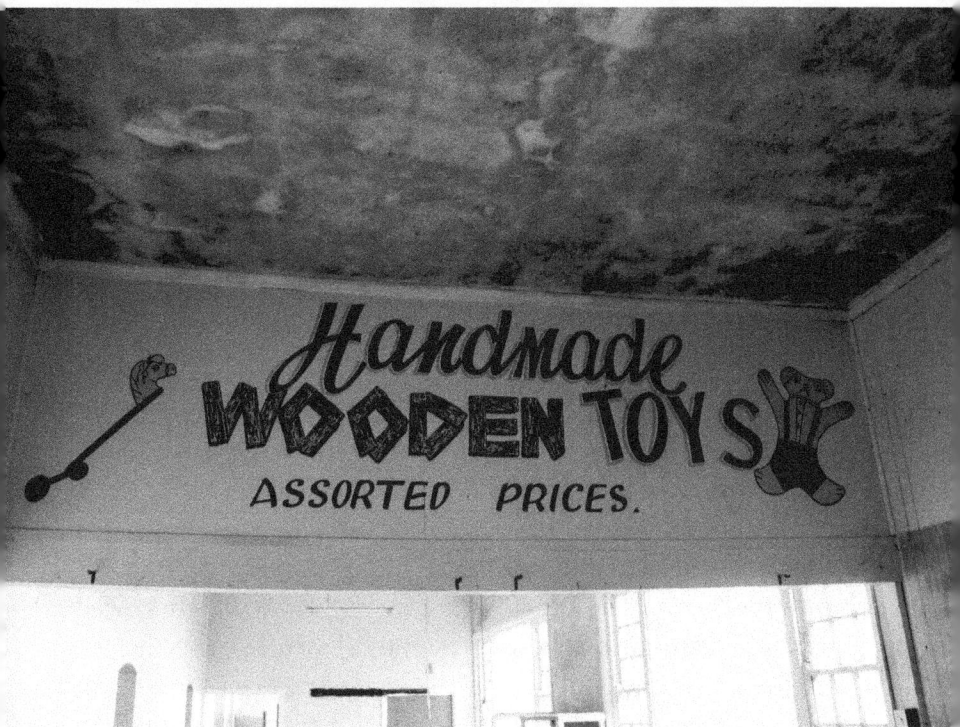

Handmade
WOODEN TOYS
ASSORTED PRICES.

---

23   William Oates, Male Warder 1882-1896. Promoted to Engineer 1896-1922.

24   William Rattray, Male Attendant, 1889-1909.

25   John Christie, Cook, 1902-1907.

preparation for the next meal. No ornamental parlor is this place, but the very hub of the local universe — the dynamo where all its vital force is generated. Everything is disposed with a view to efficiency, for even a momentary hitch in the arrangements here is a very serious matter. Sacks of potatoes, parsnips and other edibles stand conveniently about ready for the boiling process, which is all done by steam; this being considered safer, cleaner and more economical than fire.

A PATIENT AT HOME.

Mr. Banko[26], the genial head-wardsman, now comes on the scene, and I am forth-with taken over the male portion of the building. First of all there are the semi-detached cottages to see. These are arranged as nearly as possible on the plan of those on the female side. Here I am introduced to Mr. White, the artist. Mr. White is one of the oldest patients in the Asylum, and has whiled away the tedium of many long years by means of his brush, which he manipulates with much artistic precision and skill. This gentleman was good enough to take me round his studio, where I was shown some excellent work both in water-color and in oils. Mr. White has a robust taste for the realistic in art, and with much evident satisfaction produced for my inspection a careful reproduction of a picture of the crucifixion in the pre-Raphaelite style, critically observing: "You know, I don't like these modern Christs; they are such effeminate creatures." This patient is a severe sufferer from melancholia, but is all other respects appears intelligent and rational. After leaving Mr. White I met Lord Eglinton, who sorrowfully informed me in the authority of the King himself that His Majesty would be unable to pay him a visit this week — a piece of news which, I need hardly say, caused me no surprise, but at which, nevertheless, I ventured to express my regret. Then commenced the tour of the male wards and dormitories, all of which are models of cleanliness, as they are also the perfection of order. In passing along an upper corridor I got a good view of the airing courts. One of these is known as the "Refractory Court," because it is

---

26 Thomas Banko, Male Attendant, 1902-1905.

confined to the use of cases of mania. It is a rectangle enclosed in high brick walls. I remember once going through it with Dr. M'Burnie[27], a former medical officer, who wanted to demonstrate the mental condition of certain of the in mates. He had scarcely commenced to question the patients when a tall, dark-looking-giant of a fellow took it into his head that a conspiracy was going forward to imprison him for life. And I was the unfortunate principal of the plot. I shall not forget the raving manner in which lie pursued us round the yard, with a crowd of others in his wake. Never was I lashed with such Doric[28], such fierce, unmentionable barbaresque[29]! You could have heard him two miles off. Nor shall I forget the self-possessed manner in which the worthy Doctor, deluged in this flood of sound and fury, quietly gave the gaunt looking warder directions for this man's treatment, as he fumbled in his waistcoat pocket for the little key that was to let us out through the big door. I have no very strong desire to go through that yard again. I think I rather prefer to view it from up here. Mr. Banko tells me there was little real danger, because maniacs never act in a body. One madman may call on his fellows to help him to murder another, but they take no notice of him. This is a fortunate circumstance, for if it were otherwise, the number of attendants would have to be indefinitely multiplied.

THE MONOMANIAC.

The fact is many of them are mono maniacs, and are too fully occupied with their own thoughts to have much regard for those of others. Here for instance comes a pale looking, flabby faced man with wandering, watery eyes, who imagines that he is preyed upon by some unseen agency. He believes that gases are being injected into his body whilst he is asleep! There goes

---

27 Stuart MacBirnie, Medical Officer, 1897-? (at time of printing, an ending date could not be found).

28 Doric : a dialect of ancient Greek spoken in the Peloponnesus, Crete, certain of the Aegean Islands, Sicily, and southern Italy.

29 Barbaresque: stylistically barbaric.

another poor beggar who fancies that somebody is inside him, and he can't get this somebody out! Poor fellow! Here is a patient who has enormous wealth, has already paid off the national debt, and is about to build palaces and endow numerous institutions for the public good. Just let him out and see! Another is suffering from enlarged ideas — a common complaint — and supposes that he is some great orator or poet, or that he has miraculous powers and can command the sum and control the elements.

A WIDE SUBJECT.

There are so many different phases of lunacy. Indeed it is very hard to say precisely in what insanity consists. Many attempts have been made to define the word; but as the varieties of mental disease classed under the term are so numerous, and their distinctions in some cases so great, and in others so minute, medical experts themselves are unable to make a definition such as shall any practical value. All eccentric people are considered to be somewhere on the borderland, and these people are so numerous that a great European University professor has elaborately endeavored [sic] to prove that the earth itself is nothing short of a lunatic asylum; on no other hypothesis can lie account for insane things which people generally do. This confirms the contention of Boileau[30], the great French writer, who declared that all men were mad, the only difference being that some men showed more skill than others in covering up the crack. For ordinary purposes, however, the insane are divided by physicians into four classes, mania, monomania, dementia and idiocy. These again have their sub divisions and varieties almost ad infinitum. It was quite late in the afternoon when I reached the secretary's office. Here I was received by Mr. Cody[31], the new secretary, who answered some questions I had to ask concerning the general management of the institution. Mr. Cody

---

30   Boileau (French *bwalo*) Nicolas Boileau-Despréaux, French poet and critic; author of satires, epistles, and L'Art poétique (1674), in which he laid down the basic principles of French classical literature.

31   John Cody, Manager, 1903-1908.

struck me as being a very urbane[32] and intelligent officer. He has, apparently, a clear, business-like grasp of his work, and will make, in every respect, I should imagine, a worthy successor to Capt. T. Vicars Foote[33], who was for many years in charge of this department, and who is now on the retired list. I was sorry to be unable to visit the kitchen garden and the farm, both of which, I am assured, area credit to the institution. The former, which has an area of some 16 acres, is directed by Mr. Bolle[34], "whose prodigious pumpkins and other vegetables have made him locally famous. The farm is managed by Mr. Nimon[35], and is 200 acres in extent. It is, however, an indispensable adjunct, and the milk, butter, jam — of which many tons are consumed annually — and other commodities produced in abundance from it, indicate another of the many economic factors which, taken altogether, bring the working expenses of the institution, down to an average of 10s per patient per week. Dr. Samson, the superintendent, must be a very responsible man. His work, I should think, demands qualifications of the rarest kind. He must be personally benevolent and firm; humane, just and inflexible. He must have a sound and practical knowledge of human nature in all its phases, as well as infinite tact. He must also have a general knowledge of business; understand house architecture and engineering; know something of farming and gardening— for he has to supervise all the operations of the institution; he should be acquainted with various trades and manufactures. Combined with these qualifications, too, he must be skilled in his own profession in all its several departments. The onerous duties of management are shared by Dr. Rattan[36], the assistant medical officer of the institution. Doctor Samson talked to me

32 Urbane: polished and elegant in manner or style.

33 Thomas Foote, Manager, 1894-1902.

34 William Bolle, Cook , 1890-1902. Gardener 1902-? (at time of printing, an ending date could not be found).

35 Joseph Nimon, Male Attendant, 1898-1901. Farm Bailiff, 1901-1910.

36 Arthur Rattan, Medical Officer, 1901-1903.

on the subject of the treatment. This aims at the restoration of the general health, and at the removal of any local trouble, I was gratified to learn that the treatment, combined with other auxiliaries, is successful in forty per cent, of the cases admitted."

"[T]his section is easily the most historically-important part of the facility due to it still retaining the most original layout of any ward in the asylum. It is the only wing in which the early pink-hued wash finish to the external render remains visible." (*Palace of Broken Dreams*, 2017, p.23)

"The asylum building had a very austere interior and efforts were made by the staff to ameliorate the institutional atmosphere. In 1880, it was reported that the Matron of the female section at Beechworth imparted an air of 'comfort' to the wards through their decoration with curtains and antimacassars[37], and the placement of indoor plants. Three years later, paintings had been added to the walls, and 'live and stuffed birds' and animals were placed in hanging cages." (Lovell Chen, 2012, p.16)

"The neatness of the female patients was particularly noticeable, and we believe that this is in a great measure due to the attention and taste of Mrs Sharpe, the matron, who takes a pride in having her particular charges nicely dressed and

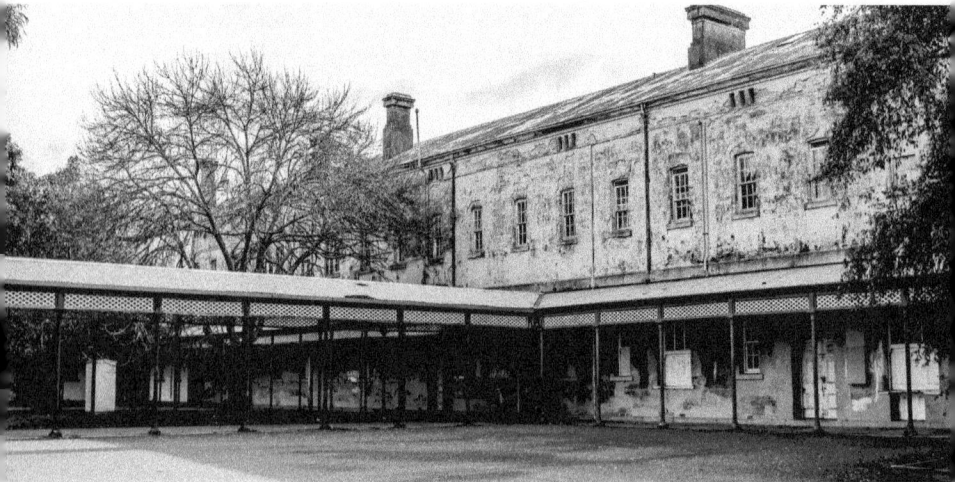

_____

37 Antimacassar: a protective and often decorative covering for the back or arms of a chair or sofa.

presentable." (*Ovens and Murray Advertiser*, Saturday 15 April 1882, p.4)

Excerpt from "Picturesque Victoria" by 'The Vagabond', *The Argus*, **Friday, 8th August, 1884, p.6**

"The female wards at the Beechworth asylum are decidedly an improvement on anything I have yet seen in Australia. There are more pictures, more ornaments and attempts at decoration. A woman, unless she is in the very worst stage, will not attempt to destroy anything pleasing to the eye. These wards would be quite a treat to the members of the Kalizoic Society[38], and I dare say would also be a lesson to many of them. There are some really bad cases here - old harridans whom drink and evil passions have destroyed, who would tear down any bird cage and rend to pieces any of the crewel work covers which we see in some of the wards. The matron is to be congratulated on the taste she displays in working these. Some of the women are of the class known as "highly dangerous". One hag makes a rush with the design to embrace me, preparatory to scratching out my eyes, but is stopped by the two stalwart young women attendants in this ward. The Chinese woman, speaking broken English as she does, is a horror. I do not know why the majority of the female lunatics here should be of the Irish race, but such is the case. The life led by a female attendant is a repulsive one, and the wonder is how any respectable young woman will take such a place. It hardens, almost unsexes, them. All pity is choked in their hearts by what they have to experience. There is however, one young girl, an attendant in the sick ward here, who has such a patient, nurse-like face that I feel inclined to take my hat off to her. I hear that her looks do not belie her appearance. She is from the German Fatherland, the country of patient women. The most distressing case I see is that of the woman, a recruit of the Salvation Army. She throws herself continually into hysteric convulsions, possessed like those of old by a devil calling on

---

38 The Kalizoic Society was formed in 1884... and... advocated a widespread 'love of the beautiful' among Melburnians.

the name of the Lord. There is anxiety in Dr. Deshon's[39] eyes as he endeavours to soothe this poor lunatic, but there is also deep sympathy. He is one who evidently feels the importance of the position he holds. This woman is more to him than a mere "case"; there is a human soul distraught by wild passions. My flinty heart, too, is touched at this sight, and back through the mist of ages my mind travels to the Syrian hills where tradition tells us the Great Healer cured those who were "sore vexed and fell into the fire and into the water", and cast out the fierce devils which possessed men. The age of miracles is past, this is a wicked and perverse generation; prayer and fasting are held to be of little avail. But sceptical though many of us may be, the Religion of Humanity preached by Him of Nazareth has had its effect in the recent rational treatment of lunatics, the influence of the Gesta Christi[40] is felt even in the Asylum.

What I particularly admire in the female wards here is the home-like appearance which, as far as possible, is imparted to the dreary corridors and dormitories. In the work-room where sewing machines are clicking and many patients are employed with needle and thread, one would hardly imagine that you were in the midst of a lunatic asylum. The same also in the laundry. When insane men and women are at work the "nor'-nor'-west" madness with which they are afflicted is kept in abeyance[41]. In this respect there is an advantage in the treatment of female lunatics over males. A woman is more accustomed to housework; is her second nature to scrub and clean, and sew. She is happy when employed in this manner. It is more difficult to provide occupation for the males. Indoors there is nothing they can do except clean out their wards – work not natural to a man and to which, as I remember at Kew, patients were sometimes driven with curses and sometimes with blows. That may be the

39 Frederick Deshon, 3rd Superintendent, 1882-1896.

40 *Gesta Christi: a History of Humane Progress Under Christianity.* Brace, Charles Loring. London: Hodder & Stoughton. 1883.

41 Abeyance: the condition of being temporarily set aside; suspension.

case here for I know very well the brutalising effect this prison barrack system has upon warders. In a few months, if I had retained my position it Kew, I daresay I too should have been hardened to the extent of occasionally "hammering", a harmless lunatic – on the back of the neck be it understood, where the blows would leave little mark, or could be accounted for to the doctor as the result of a fall. But if female lunatics can be advantageously employed inside, the males, per contra[42], can be utilised in outdoor work. Free exercise and fresh air are powerful antidotes to evil spirits. In the 200 acres reserve attached to the Beechworth Asylum many patients are employed under the supervision of the bailiff. They are certainly in far better case than those who can only take exercise inside the sunken walls which surround the asylum. There are 20 acres under different crops of vegetables, and there is also a fine fruit garden. Besides home consumption the hospital and Benevolent Asylum are supplied with garden produce. The cows, which roam through the uncleared paddocks, afford milk to the institution. I am called upon to admire these as well as the pigs and the poultry which are being fattened for sale in Beechworth. After inspecting the farm buildings, I leave this institution, pleased that everything possible is apparently done for the humane care of the patients, but more than ever impressed with the idea that the principle upon which the lunatic asylums of Victoria are conducted is one to be deprecated. Exception is made in favour of Yarra Bend, but that is to be sapiently[43] broken up."

"Patients who were capable of helping performed many duties associated with the care and delivery of all the laundered material for the entire asylum: washing, drying, ironing, folding and storage of clothes, linen and blankets all took place in the Laundry.

The double-height ceiling and vent system allowed for the extremely hot and moist atmosphere of the working laundry processes." (*Palace of Broken Dreams*, 2017, p.28)

---

42 Per contra: On the contrary; by way of contrast.
43 Sapiently: having great wisdom and discernment.

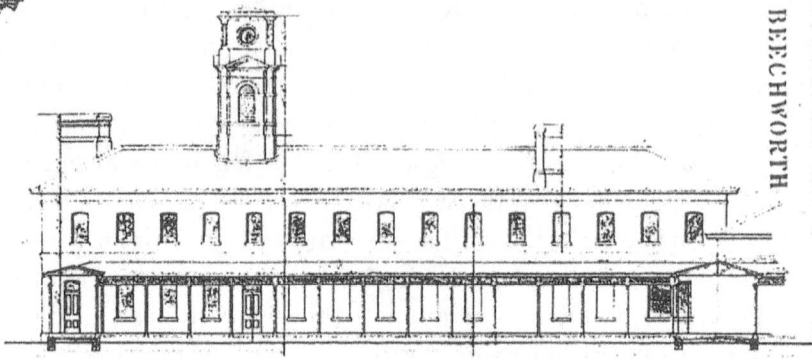

SIDE ELEVATION

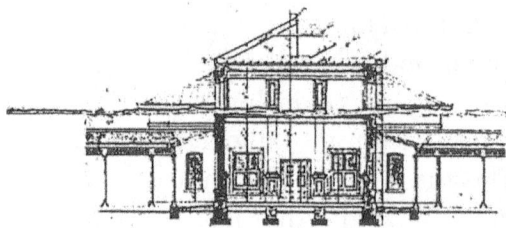

SECTION C.D.

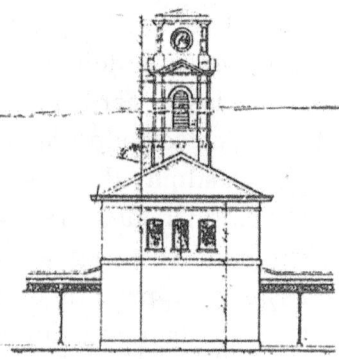

END ELEVATION

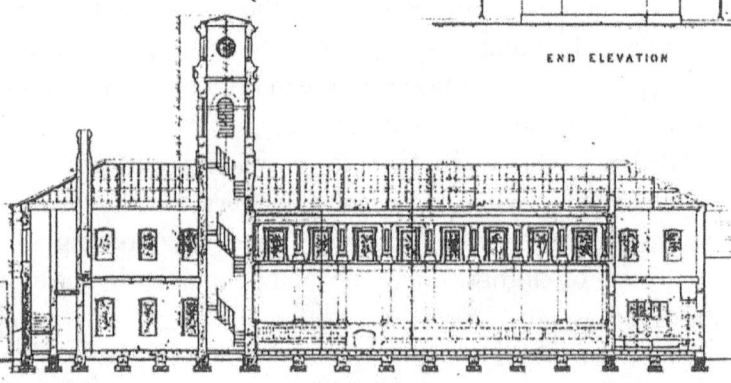

SECTION A.B.

The hall – Bijou Theatre – was constructed between 1864-67 and forms a part of the asylum core. When viewed from overhead, it forms the centre stroke of a capital E.

Bijou is French for little jewel and, in later years, bijou was used to describe a charming building. It was used for recreation, special events, church services, and dances. It housed two reading rooms and the entrance to the bell tower. Upstairs there was a billiard room which later became a pharmacy.

"Most of the 'amusements' were held at the institution itself and involved staff and patients, but the ongoing involvement of the local Beechworth community is noteworthy. A mixture of entertainment and sport was offered. For example, in 1890, the amusements for the year comprised two fancy dress balls, five minstrel performances by the staff and a range of sporting activities. In addition, many of the patients who were able, attended local races and other sporting events, with the support of the local residents. A bowling green was established as early as the 1870s, and a library was stocked with books for use by the patients." (Lovell Chen, 2012, p.15)

"The stores area in the east end of the wing comprises two large store rooms on the ground floor and rooms to the north and south originally used as female and male attendants' mess rooms respectively." (*Palace of Broken Dreams*, 2017, p.14)

All supplies – meat, eggs, vegetables, fruit, linen, clothes, etc. would have been brought in through these doors and stored in various rooms including the cellar.

"The cellar below the stores was the cold-storage area for meats and other perishables. It takes up the same area below ground level as the stores area does above." (*Palace of Broken Dreams*, 2017, p.17)

THE INFIRMARY

"This building was constructed in 1889-90 as two 14-patient cottages for male patients comprising an attendant room, store, two wards, a day room and single cells laid out in a U-shape. The buildings were linked at the rear (west side) by verandahs and a shared bathroom and kitchen pavilion.

Alterations and additions in 1913-14 involved the construction of a new dormitory between the two buildings to create a large central dormitory which joined the cottages and created a small open court between the new dormitory and the bathroom and kitchen pavilion. Substantial alterations and additions in 1959 comprised the construction of utility rooms in the open court, the enclosing of the verandahs along the west elevation to form corridors, the construction of a dining room and day room extension at the north end of the north cottage as well as additionalbathroom and laundry facilities at the south end of the south cottage." (*Palace of Broken Dreams*, 2017, p.39-40)

CHWORTH ASYLUM

WO COTTAGES FOR m PATIENTS EACH

Scale 1/16 ... 1 inch

MALE SIDE

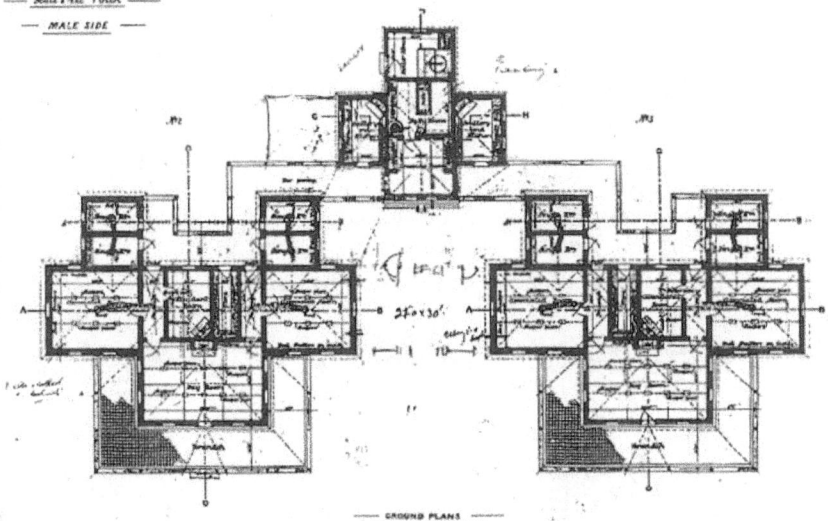

GROUND PLANS

MNS-2.345

BEECHWORTH
ASYLUM FOR INSANE

NEW DORMITORY BETWEEN COTTAGES Nos 1&3 MALE SIDE
SCALE 8 FT = 1 INCH

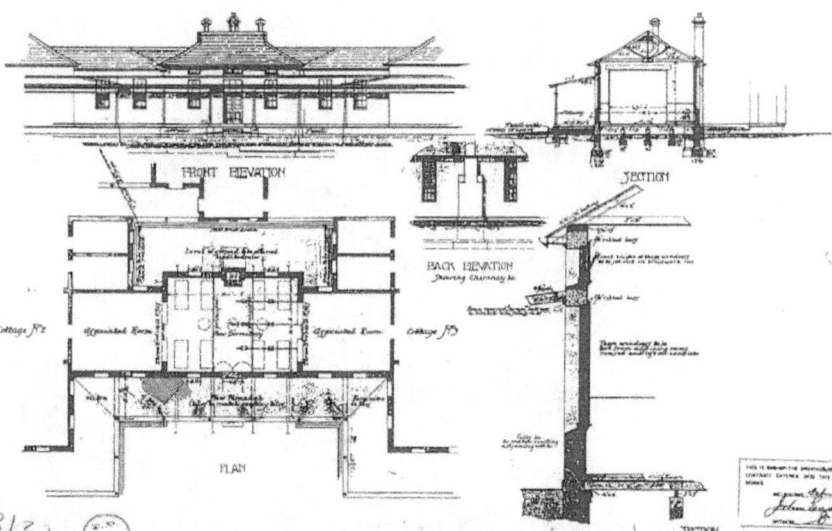

FRONT ELEVATION

SECTION

BACK ELEVATION
Showing Chimneys &c

PLAN

Cottage No 2   Associated Room   Associated Room   Cottage No 3

SECTION

HOSPITAL FOR THE INSANE

BEECHWORTH

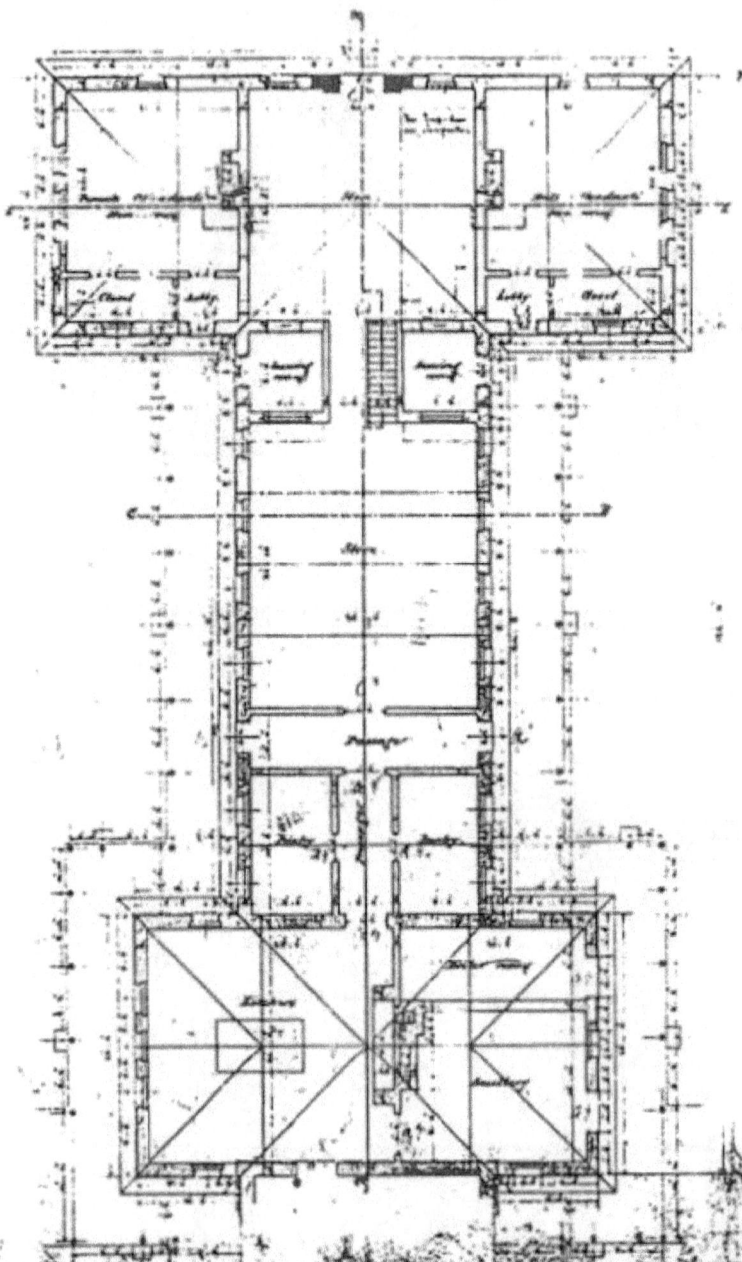

GROUND PLAN

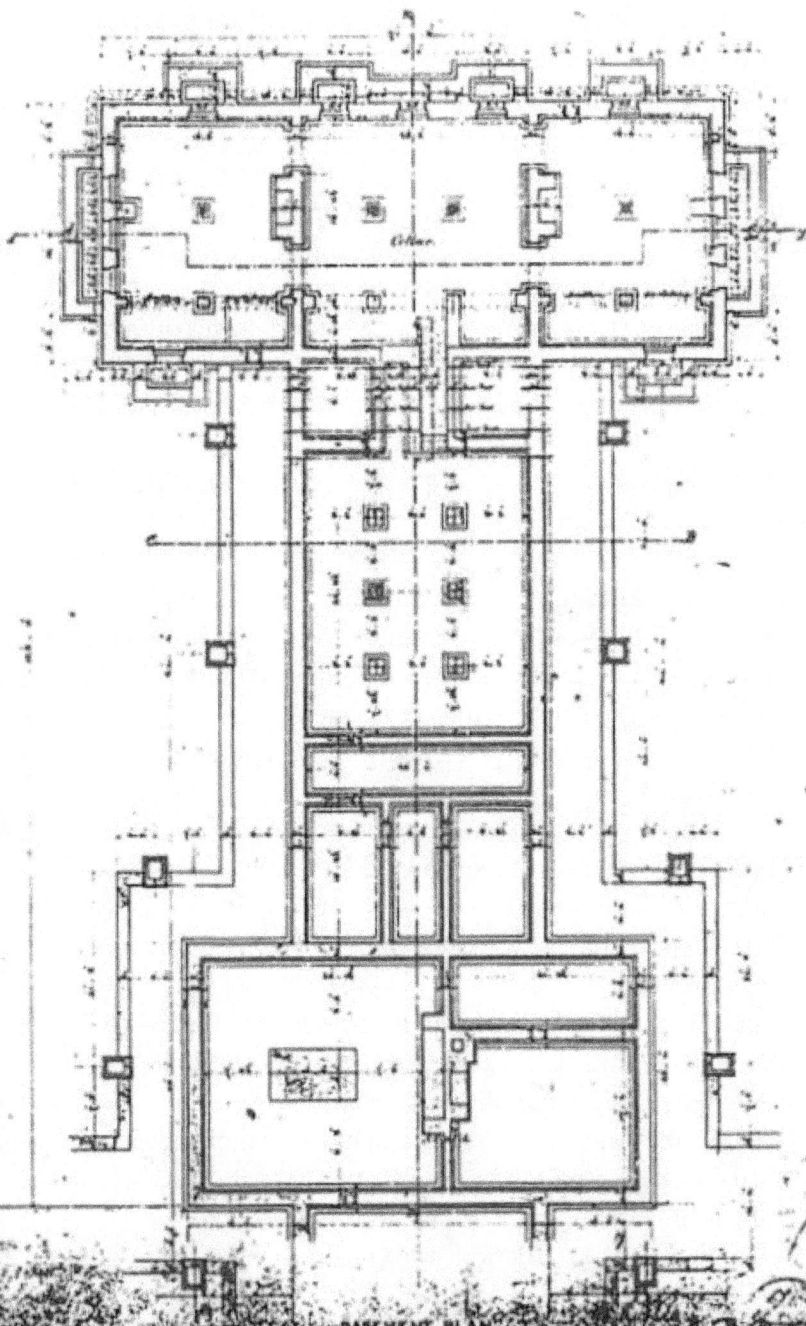

BASEMENT PLAN

Beechworth Asylum time line

1864 — A site was selected and building commenced.

1867 — Beechworth Lunatic Asylum opened for 250 patients.

1870 — The Ha-Ha Wall and front Gatehouse (group accommodation) were built.

1872 — Male extension wing was added to accommodate an additional 88 patients (Sapphire and Garnet/'Bullpit') and female extension wing to accommodate 50 patients (demolished 1976).

1872 — Medical Officer's Quarters was built (McCarthy House/private residence).

1872 — Stables were built.

1877 — Gas lighting was introduced.

1878 — Outside roundhouses/rotundas were constructed in the airing courts to provide shelter for inmates (demolished).

1886 — Gas lighting replaced kerosene.

1889 — Cottage wards were built: four on male side (Olivene, Grevillea, Kurrajong) and four on the female side (Carinya, Myrtle/Kiama).

1902 — One female cottage ward was converted to a hospital and infirmary (demolished 1971).

1902 — Two cottages were joined on male side to form a hospital (Grevillea).

1905 — Renamed Beechworth Hospital for the Insane.

1907 — Male and female mess rooms were built (Kiosk on male side/female side demolished 1980s).

1907 — Superintendent's residence built (demolished).

1910 — Cricket pavilion built.

1913 — Butcher complex built. Extended 1947.

1914 — Hot water radiation introduced to heat some of the female wards.

1926—Electricity was connected.

1934—Renamed Beechworth Mental Hospital.

1937—Nurses Home built (Linaker Hotel).

1938—First ward built outside the Ha-Ha Wall to take excess patients (children) from Kew Cottages – (Turquoise/The Pines/ Indigo Shire Offices).

1938—Water sewerage system connected.

1939—Projection equipment was installed to run movies in Bijou Theatre as part of recreation program.

1951—Large section of male side was destroyed by a fire.

1951—Original slate roof was replaced by tin (some slate tiles were used to house the butchers).

1951—Extensions made to Nurses Home.

1954 —Fire damaged wards were renovated.

1954—Modern drugs and the 'Open Door' policy were introduced for patient management.

1955—Bell Tower on the Bijou Theatre was demolished.

1957 —Demolition of the Ha-Ha Wall commenced due to the 'Open Door' policy.

1959—Boiler House built.

1959—New Morgue was built (demolished).

1964—Became a nurse training centre.

1967—Engineer's workshops (Madman's Gully Wines) built.

1970—Renamed Beechworth Mental Hospital.

1974 —Female wing adjacent to the laundry was abandoned.

1976—George Kerferd Clinic was built (George Kerferd Hotel). Built on the site of the superintendent's residence.

1976—Two psychogeriatric wards were built (Amethyst and Emerald/Beechworth Fitness).

1976 —Female wing extension was demolished.

1978—Original Mortuary converted and consecrated to become the Chapel of the Resurrection.

1979—Front female wing renovated into Nurses Training School and Occupational Therapy Unit.

1980—Laundry shutdown and services were outsourced – laundry and adjacent female wing used for storage.

1981—Regothermic kitchen complex built (Beechworth Storage).

1995—Beechworth Psychiatric Hospital was decommissioned.

1996 —La Trobe University purchased the site.

2015—Mayday Hills Pty Ltd purchased the site.

2015—Subdivisions commenced.

2015 —Asylum Ghost Tours – Beechworth purchsed buildings and started trading.

List of Superintendents

1867-1877—Dick, Thomas Thomson
1877-1882—Watkins, William L
1882-1896—Deshon, Frederick
1896-1905—Samson, Henry
1905-1912—Philpott, Alfred
1912-1915—Hollow, Joseph
1915-1922—Catarinich, John
1922-1929—Naylor, Rupert George St John
1929-1932—Cade, David Duncan
1932-1933—Curtis, Albert
1933-1937—Rogers, James Sydney Alexander
1937-1940—Ryan, William Bernard
1940-1942—Ridge, Clive Farran
1942-1945—Retallick, Thomas Grenville C
1945-1946—Edmonds, Horace Joseph Carlyle
1946-1951—Stone, Harold Crowcombe
1951-1952—Roberts, Edgar Lennard
1952-1954—Goding, Geoffrey Arthur
1954-1956—Bower, Herbert Michael
1956-1956—Fordyce, John Leys
1956-1963—Donnan, Laurence Frederick
1963-1967—Burt, Cyril Gavin
1967-1970—Jensen, Graeme
1970-1976—Whitaker, Howard L
1976-1977—Darby, Edward J
1977-1983—Mason, John L
1983-1988—West, Rosemary
1988—Position of Superintendent became redundant

LIST OF MATRONS

1867-1872—Dunne, Bridget
1872-1878—McGuire, Maria
1879-1893—Sharp, Elizabeth
1893-1895—Kilkelly, Catherine
1895-1901—Holland, Mary
1901-1903—No permanent appointment
1903-1905—Cameron, Mary McN
1905-1907—Richardson, Ada F
1907-1923—Short, Maria
1925-1927—Puddiphatt, Mary E
1927-1935—Beckmann, Eda P
1936-1937—Couch, Bridget
1937-1938—Stanley, Eileen D
1938-1942—Larsen, Malvina
1942-1953—McGrath, Mary E
1953-1955—Carter Christina (acting)
1955-1959—Evans, Susannah
1959-1967—Fanning, Mary I
1967-1976—McDonald, Eva M (position changed to Director of Nursing in 1975)

References

"A Run Through Beechworth Lunatic Asylum". *Ovens and Murray Advertiser*. 6th June, 1903. p.11.

"Beechworth Lunatic Asylum Historic Dates". La Trobe at Beechworth, 1997.

"Conservation Management Plan Review". East Melbourne: Lovell Chen, 2012.

D.A. Craig. *The Lion of Beechworth: An Account of the Mayday Hills Hospital, Beechworth*. Thurgoona: Specialty Press, 2000.

Find My Past. "Find Your Ancestors in Victoria, Mental Health Institutions".

Finn, Rev. William Mason. *Glimpses of North-Easter Victoria, and Albury, New South Wales,* Chapter 10. pp. 24-26. Catholic Bookselling and Printing Depot: Melbourne, 1870.

Palace of Broken Dreams: A Brief History of Beechworth Asylum. Beechworth: Asylum Ghost Tours – Beechworth, 2017.

"The Beechworth Lunatic Asylum". *Ovens and Murray Advertiser: Supplement to the Ovens and Murray Advertiser*. 23rd May 1867. p.1.

The Free Dictionary. www.thefreedictionaty.com

'The Vagabond'. "Picturesque Victoria". *The Argus*. 8th August 1884. p.6

Trove. National Library of Australia. https://trove.nla.gov.au

Zox Commission/ Royal Commission on Asylums for the Insane and Inebriates 1884 – 1886.

LIST OF PLACES TO START YOUR ASYLUM RESEARCH

Anne Hanson, Family & Social Historian (Beechworth Historian & Researcher). https://sites.google.com/site/annehansonfamilyhistory

Archival Access Victoria (Research and digitisation of Victoria's archival records). https://www.archivalaccessvictoria.com or https://www.facebook.com/ArchivalAccessVictoria

Beechworth Cemetery Trust. https://www.beechworthcemetery.com.au

D.A. Craig. *The Lion of Beechworth: An Account of the Mayday Hills Hospital, Beechworth.* Thurgoona: Specialty Press, 2000.

Find and Connect (Australian orphanages, children's Homes and other institutions). https://www.findandconnect.gov.au

Find My Past. https://www.findmypast.com.au

Palace of Broken Dreams: A Brief History of Beechworth Asylum. Beechworth: Asylum Ghost Tours - Beechworth, 2017.

Public Records Office of Victoria. State Government of Victoria (PROV). https://www.prov.vic.gov.au

Trove. National Library of Australia (digitised copies of old newspapers, journals, magazines, books, photos). https://trove.nla.gov.au

Victorian Government Gazette: Online Archive 1836-1997. State Library of Victoria. http://gazette.slv.vic.gov.au

* 9 7 8 1 9 2 5 6 2 3 3 9 0 *